Baby and Beyond: Natural, Healthy Loving Care

Dr. Elvis Ali, ND

ISBN: 153914710X
ISBN-13: 9781539147107

DISCLAIMER

The information in this book are at all times restricted to education, teaching and training on the subject of natural health matters intended for general natural health well-being and do not involve the diagnosing, prognosticating, treatment, or prescribing of remedies for the treatment of any disease, or any licensed or controlled act which may constitute the practice of medicine.

Questions? Contact us at: **drelvisali10@hotmail.com**

CONTENTS

ACKNOWLEDGMENTS

It is a pleasure to acknowledge with thanks:

My entire family in Canada and Trinidad and Tobago who have continued to support and motivate me to educate others about naturopathic medicine. My parents, Hakim, Hazrah, my sisters, Alima, Homaida, Homeeda, Fazida, my children, Hassan, Azeeda, Kareem, nephews, nieces and precious grandchildren, Gursimran, Meheirveer and Shairveer for their encouragement and belief in holistic medicine.

Colleagues in the health care profession, especially Dr. Leo Roy.

My students and staff at CCNM, BINM, CCHH, OAND, CAND and clinics, BTNL, AA Comfort Health Centers and Mississauga clinic. The companies for their assistance in educating the public about preventative medicine: Biorrific, Ecoideas, Canadian Bio, Sangsters, Fion Beauty Supplies Canada, Alpha Science Laboratories – A division of Omega Alpha Pharmaceuticals Inc.

My dear friends, Bonita, Pat, Roy, Cindy and Darryl, Janak, Joan, Ash and Harry, Saira and Moe Sheikh from Etobicoke Motors, along with many others too numerous to list.

My publisher and editor Sherree and Lillian who designed the book cover.

Having a child means...

Tender Loving Care

Total Loving Care

Total Nutrition Care

Tender Emotional Care

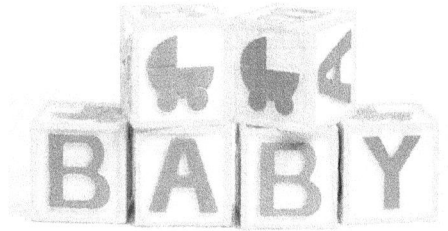

INTRODUCTION

If anyone needs and deserves perfect health and top priority are our children. They are the future of humankind. To give a child anything but the best healthcare and most nutritious foods, and to provide anything but the most favorable and harmonious surroundings, seems inconceivable. Tampering with anything of God's nature only destroys and tears to pieces the bodies, bones, teeth and the blood of our children. To tamper only inhibits the potential of one of God's masterpieces.

TLC (total loving care) is positive, warm affections: touching, holding, caressing and talking to your child. Everything that goes into and contacts the baby's body and mind, even colors and harmonious sounds will affect the baby throughout its whole life.

Only pure water and air; completely natural, alive, fresh, untreated, and unpolluted foods are intended as foods for adults and children. Clean fresh unpolluted air, natural light is indispensable, irreplaceable sustainers of life.

The first seven years determines the nature of the child for the rest of his/her life. A child's nature and potential as a fine, personable, lovable, intelligent and beautiful human being will be as great as the quality of foods, affection and environment they will live in.

"DIET is an absolutely necessary pre-condition of life and health." – Prof. Katase.

~~~

"Perfect health comprises perfect form and structure of the body, perfect functioning of the organs and of the body as a whole, maximum immunity from infection and an astonishing power of recuperation after injuries."– Dr. Bircher-Benner

~~~

"The ideal of health consists in the ability of each individual organ of the body to be equal in a high degree, at any time, to the demands which are made on it." – Prof. Marti Sigle of Riga.

~~~

The main development during the first six months of a baby's life is the brain. All substances that enter the blood stream go first to the brain. Substances that do not provide the exact and complete needs for brain growth and health are 'abnormal'.

Abnormal foods, chemicals and drugs retard brain development, alter behavioral patterns create anxieties, aggressiveness, hyperactivity and destructiveness. They have an impact on your baby's future personality and living.

Diet is the controlling influence of life and health. To create vitality and sustain the whole person, all foods must be taken in a state similar to the original state they existed in nature: unhampered with untreated, unadulterated or artificially preserved, or destroyed by chemicals, cooking, microwaves or radiations. A parent's care, love and attention, together with mother's milk provide a baby's total needs.

Our busy, modern lifestyle and commercial enterprises have conditioned parents to replace love with comforts and conveniences, and convenient foods. The chemical and food industries have seduced parents to forfeit the life-regenerating values of natural, chemically free, wholesome, alive foods with those that are devitalized, embalmed and denatured. It is a tragedy.

Taking the time to nurture your baby with good quality wholesome foods will pay off in the years to come.

This "back to basics" book will empower you to make the right healthy choices for your baby's health and wellbeing. However, it is also very wise to work in partnership with your pediatrician. Consult with him or her on the choices you would like to make for your baby. It's important that both of you want the best outcome for the child.

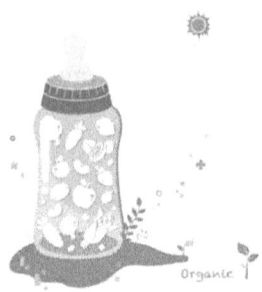

1 MOTHER'S VERSUS COW'S MILK

Mother's milk is the only food that provides all the life forces, balance, health and healing. Babies and children need everything they can get to be and grow well.

Every poor quality food deprives your baby of needed essentials. Training a child's taste and appetite for foods of inferior quality may turn a child against patterns of eating that affect optimal living throughout his/her life. The other nutrients of cows or goat's milk do not provide a child's needs in the same perfect balance as does mother's milk. Only mother's milk contains all the specific nutrients required for the growth of the mind and nervous system.

It is important to realize and accept that milk, and especially cow's milk, is not essential to the health of babies (or to anyone), as common opinion and the dairy industries would have us believe. It is preferable not to use animal milk. It is meant for animals.

The hormones that are in mother's milk perfectly provide for and balance all the body's need for a baby's slow, steady growth. The amount of hormones in cow's milk is extremely excessive. They activate a growth of up to six hundred pounds in the first year of a calf. Inordinate growth in an infant (and in adults), can somewhat weaken its constitution for its future lifetime. Since growth of the infant slows down at the age of two years, it becomes all the more important that the growth-promoting stimuli of cow's milk be left aside.

The requirements of the organisms are changed. The body's reserve of iron that comes naturally at birth is now depleted. Cow's milk does not satisfy this need.

Animal milk promotes premature lankiness of growth, abnormal rise in body temperature and early teeth decay. Children, so fed, have increased susceptibility to diseases of all kinds.

Mother's milk contains immunity factors and elements that provide a strong protection against common diseases, bowel and respiratory infections, and many other infant infections and diseases. These are not found in cow's milk. Cow's milk is lacking in the oils and fats that are essential to a baby's needs. Stomachs of babies have difficulties digesting animal milks. Cow's milk is more difficult to digest and assimilate than goat's milk. Cows have four stomachs for digesting their foods.

Animals never touch their mothers' milk after they are weaned, except the two-legged ones. This is a lesson we need to learn from nature. Once a baby has been weaned from the breast, it is not advisable to feed it milk, especially an animal's milk.

The nutrients required for a child are radically different from those of a cow. They contain fewer proteins. The difference in composition, and the balance of its components, make cow's milk an unsatisfactory substitute for the milk of the mother. Even diluting it with water and adding a good source of honey is inadequate. Infant disorders still result from feedings with cow's milk.

With cow's milk as a child's sole food, all too soon they become sickly.

Breast Feeding

Never deprive a baby of the benefits of breast feeding. Provide the baby with mother's milk for as long as possible. The breast-fed infant becomes a better adjusted child and adult, because he/she had been held and loved, and made to feel secure while being fed. The baby will develop a better formation of facial structure, because of the sucking and the facial muscle action involved.

Problems arise when a mother cannot breast feed right from the beginning and when a pediatrician's stereotyped 'formula' fails to replace nutrients provided by breast milk. However, there are alternate ways of feeding that make available all essential nutrients. They eliminate the hazards of toxic, artificial and wrong foods. They help prevent childhood diseases. They greatly help to create a child that is happy, playful and eager to learn, and above all, very healthy.

WAYS TO INCREASE MILK PRODUCTION

- Get plenty of rest. Whenever possible, nap frequently during the day.
- Maintain an attitude of a calm, accepting, peaceful approach towards everything, while nursing your baby.
- Drink lots of hot water and herb teas, such as clover tea.
- Use lots of sprouts, such as alfalfa.
- Use whole grains, especially corn, millet, flax seed and sesame seed, milled and served as a breakfast cereal, and/or mixed with oatmeal porridge.
- Use generous amounts of sesame and sunflower seeds in raw salads.
- Use yeasts, especially the live forms, such as Fleischmann's yeast. Also brewer 's yeast in a superior concentrate form of Vitamin B complex.

Supplements: Pituitary extracts (protomorphogens) Biost powder (Standard process laboratories), Choline in food concentrate tablets or Fortil B-12 .

PASTEURIZED MILK

The food babies have the greatest difficulty tolerating is heated (pasteurized) cow's milk. Always avoid canned, powdered and pasteurized forms of milk, including goat's milk in these forms. The worst milks are the canned, concentrated kinds.

Pasteurization destroys...

- All of the milk enzymes and almost all vitamins. Enzymes are the agents of all healing, living, immunity, feelings, thinking and body activity. Vitamins are the activators of enzymes.
- **Lecithin.** Heat disintegrates phosphoric acid and its combination with special body fats. These are called phospholipids. Phospholipids are a most essential nutrient for nerves, relaxation and resistance against viruses.
- **Casein.** Heat changes casein in milk into caseinate. Caseinate binds itself to the total milk calcium, making it non-absorbable into our tissues and unusable. Quantities of caseinate still remain unbound after taking up all the calcium. This unbound caseinate then binds with calcium in our body and prevents our body from using it. This can create a serious health problem. Calcium is essential for a multitude of body functions.
- **Milk calcium.** Heating milk transforms its calcium into an insoluble, unusable form.
- **Lactose.** A form of milk sugar. Heat caramelizes it and makes it unusable. Lactose is an essential component of the outer coating of nerves and makes up its protective sheath. It is absolutely essential to the health of nerves.

Lactose is the most favorable sugar for baby foods and it promotes the assimilation of calcium.
 Milk fats are altered.

- **Antibiotics and bactericides**. These are destroyed.
- **Citric acid and carbonic of milk**. Heat destroys them.
- **Proteins**. Up to 90 percent are denatured, perverted, destroyed and rendered unacceptable and unusable.

Overheated pasteurized milk contributes to and/or causes:

- Constipation.
- Fevers, colds, tonsillitis and swollen glands.
- Mucus and phlegm, which can accumulate, stagnate and create bronchitis, pneumonia.
- Loss of teeth and cavities.
- Predisposes to arthritis.
- Predisposes to homosexuality.
- Contributes to liver disease.
- A predisposition to cancer. Denatured proteins are toxic and favor the growth of cancer cells.
- In some babies, it causes tetany by blocking the body's availability of calcium. Vitamin B6 can prevent it.

Overheated pasteurized milk binds and immobilizes calcium that is necessary for bowel muscle relaxation, and nerve stimulation of the intestinal muscles. Muscles and nerves are deprived of it.

Note: Condensed milk creates the same effects, but to a greater degree than pasteurized milk or overheated protein foods.

MILK SUBSTITUTES

Milk substitutes provide nutrients and digestibility more valuable than animal milks. Made in the following ways, they can be almost perfect foods:

Almond, Sesame and/or Coconut Milks

- A handful of almonds
  - ½ - ¾ tsp per 8Oz feeding of sesame seeds

  and/or

- A handful of coconut cut into chunks

  and/or

- One third the quantity of each, mixed together

For each formula equivalent to an 8Oz bottle, add:

- 1-2 teaspoons of unpasteurized honey
- ¼ tablet of bee pollen or
- A pinch of Greens powder

Put them into a coffee mill/seed type blender.

- Infants don't digest foods perfectly unless crushed into minute particles.
- When grounded into a fine powder, put into a blender.
- Add a little water.
- Blend at a high speed until mixture is thick like a paste.
- Add about 1 cup of hot water. Dilute the mixture to a consistency similar to that of ordinary milk.

The above recipe prepares enough for one-to-two baby feedings.

Soy flour in small quantities, or water in which potato skins have been simmered and soaked, can be added to the nut or seed milk. They provide good proteins. Adding arrowroot flour provides a source of calcium as rich as milk. Oats, barley rice are calcium.

If there is still some sediment or granules, let the 'milk' settle. Pour off the thin liquid. Or put everything through a sieve or cheese cloth. Don't throw the solids away. Nut chunks and granules are delicious eaten on cereals.

These 'milks' are excellent. They are tastier than cow's milk and they can be used separately or in any desired combination.

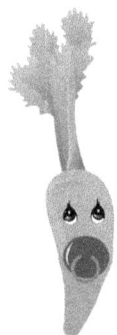

2 SELECTING & PREPARING FOODS

The first rule: food variety

Variety is important. Restricting a diet to the same foods all the time, risks creating a lack of essential nutrients. No one food supplies the baby's body with their every need.

Variety may be the only way that the body can be assured of obtaining the total and balance of all nutritional requirements, and providing all the baby's needs. Variety is important to sustain infant interests in foods.

Eggs

Range fed, fertilized eggs are top quality foods. However, incorrect feeding of hens and the diseases that affect them, markedly upset their nutritional value. Even eggs of good quality, increase putrefaction in the bowels, if and when there is any problem digesting them. They should be used with caution, if eggs are not healthy.

Cereals

Until the baby is age two, use only oats, rice and barley. These are best purchased whole and un-milled. Grind them in the blender or in a coffee mill at the time of their use. This preserves the life forces and the quality of the oils in the seeds. Rolled oats (old fashioned kind, not the quick instant oats) are excellent. They contain their own built-in anti-rancidity factors to prevent their deterioration and staleness, and rancidity of their oils.

A mixture of cereals, grains and seeds can be prepared, and used in place of, and the same as, the Pablum type or other baby cereals. After a year, sunflower seeds can be added to the above. At age two, blend and add sesame and flax seeds.

Prepare cereals by soaking them the night before using them in spring or 'mineral water'. Bring the cereal to a boil. Take the pot off the stove. Cover the pot with a lid and let the cereal, in this way, steep and cook in its own heat, overnight. Heat just before using in the morning; add honey, unsalted butter or the almond or other type of milk substitute. For superb flavor, add finely ground flax and sesame seed.

Optional: Grind up caraway seed and amaranth seeds with the flax/sesame seeds. Add: nut or almond milk, or unsweetened butter, raisins, sunflower seeds, shredded coconut, dates or similar foods according to your taste. Honey (instead of sugar – even brown sugar); cinnamon, sea salt, nutmeg, or spice of your taste.

This cereal is good for children from the second year onward. If finely milled, use from the seventh month on. It is good for constipation, fevers, and digestive disorders.

> ## Muesli or Raw Fruit Porridge
>
> This is a mixture of:
>
> Oatmeal: 2 tablespoons, soaked in water for 12 hours
>
> Add chopped or grated fruit – mashed berries, apples
>
> Use juice of ½ a fresh squeezed lemon
>
> Honey from the hive; add to suit your taste
>
> Nuts: almonds, hazel nuts and one tablespoonful, milled.

Honey (Unpasteurized only)

Infants need a generous amount of honey. It is almost a complete and perfect food. It has to be complete, if bees can live on it alone.

Children's needs for energy foods increase as they age and become more active.

Honey's nutrient value is greater than just a sweetener. It can provide the equivalent value of a good lunch.

Honey is a good sedative. It helps babies to sleep. It is a good laxative. Honey and molasses are excellent for infant constipation. Always add enough to the daily diet to maintain at least three bowel movements a day. Vary the amount until the amount of elimination is controlled and normal. Excessive intakes may cause some loose bowels or diarrhea.

Honey can be used on a nipple or on a spoon, or mixed in any food or beverage: soups, salads or cereals. To make solid honey liquid, set it in a basin of warm water and add three tablespoons of water per pound.

Molasses and maple syrup are good substitutes. Unfortunately, the high heat used in the preparation of them destroys many of their enzymes.

Quality Oils

Oils are most essential nutrients. Infants need more oils than adults. Oils are the raw materials from which the body create hormones. Hormones are the governors of all body functions, of growth and of body biochemical balance. Oils are like suits of armor that coat and protect every cell from toxic hazards and harm.

The best food-form oils and sources of oils are:

- Avocados, sesame, sunflower and flax seeds
- Whole grains and seeds
- Nuts in shells (almonds and filberts) and their oils
- The livers of fish and animals. Cod or halibut liver oils are excellent and should be a regular part of the daily intake.

Quality Proteins

Proteins, combined with calcium and other minerals, are the building materials of tissues, bones, teeth and nerves. They are the raw ingredients from which enzymes, hormones and all the growth, building and function-sustaining biochemical of our bodies are created.

After breast milk, the better sources of quality proteins for infants are:

Almonds	Carob Powder
Amaranth	Hazel Nuts
Barley	Liver
Bone Marrow	Potatoes
Brown Rice	Range-fed Eggs
Coconuts	Sesame Seeds

Soy beans, their flour and milk are a high quantity, low quality protein and should be used sparingly. If taken with other protein foods (those above), the combination becomes a balanced and good quality protein. Potato skins are high balanced and good quality protein. Potato skins are an inexpensive, high quality source of protein.

"As babies grow and become more active, extra protein becomes more and more needed and valuable to their health. For human beings, a surplus of protein intake means their subjection to chronic acidosis." - Prof Katase

Meats

Meat is also a high quantity of protein, but not a quality one. Especially the flesh meats are not essential to health as is commonly believed. Meats, milk, cheeses, refined sugar and wheat are not needed to complete and balance a diet.

The longer meats are withheld from the baby's diet, the better. If meats are to be included in the diet, the best choices are the internal organs.

They must be from healthy and naturally raised animals. If used as an infant food, the best way to benefit from flesh meats is by scraping the surface of the meat and feeding just the meat juices. This juice can be mixed with vegetable juices or other foods.

Meats and high concentrate proteins are nervous system stimulants. Children thrive better on a meatless diet that is otherwise rich in vegetables, fruits, grains, nuts and natural foods. They grow at a normal rate and display greater resistance to infection.

Meats excite the body. Especially during years of growth, meat excesses give rise to disturbances of health. They are conducive to some allergies.

Note: All pork and scavenger meats, birds, fish should not be considered as foods and should be avoided.

Gelatin

Use only natural gelatins to which no coloring, chemicals or additives have been added. They are no longer available at grocery stores, but you can purchase them from health food stores.

You can color or flavor gelatins by adding fruits or juices. **Note:** Jello is up to 53 percent sugar and loaded with artificial colorings and flavorings. Avoid!

Nuts

They are best when shelled by you and taken fresh from their shells. If purchased without shells, the skins should be intact. Air contact rancidifies the oils of exposed nuts, grains and seeds. Peanuts, slightly roasted in their shells, or peanuts freshly shelled and grounded into peanut butter are excellent foods. Strictly avoid commercial brands and hydrogenated peanut butters.

Bananas

Bananas, when naturally ripened (not smoke ripened as most commercial ones are), are excellent baby food. As soon as solid foods can be included in a baby's diet, bananas are a good food to use as a starter. Later, at six months or so, mixing bananas with peanut butter is an excellent, nutritious and quite complete meal.

Coconuts

The sweet water from a ripe coconut has a nutritional value comparable to that of quality milk. It is an excellent milk substitute. Coconut, fresh from its shell and shredded in a blender, is delicious with cereals.

Coconuts can be mixed with almonds, sesame seeds or soy flour to make a delicious and nutritious 'milk' drink. (See the preparation of almond milk above).

Mineral Rich Waters

Prepare them by simmering at low temperatures, the skins of akin foods: potatoes, root vegetables, barley, brown rice, meats, carrots, etc.

Milk substitute and soups are best made by using this kind of water. To replace minerals, lost by subjecting water to distilling or reverse osmosis, add a teaspoon of crude natural sea salt to each gallon.

Sea Salt

Use generously. Children need a lot of sea salt – as much as adults need – sometimes more. Parents tend to gauge the needs of infants by their own needs, taste or personal beliefs. Medics and media warn us against commercial table salt with reason, for it is generally made chemically and is a drug.

Sea salt is the blood of the ocean. Its formula is identical to that of human body; however, the concentration is different. Its more than 100 minerals and trace minerals are essential to growth, health and to all the functions of the human body. These elements are all in a perfect balance and in perfect harmony with the blood and body biochemistry.

The stomach, liver, kidneys, adrenal glands and brain cannot function without salt. Sea salt is healing and strengthening. Sea salt can be the only way of replenishing lack trace elements. They are critical to life.

Minerals and trace minerals are not available in most commercial foods. Chemical fertilizers do not restore minerals to the soil. Foods grown on chemically fertilized soil are mineral deficient.

Fresh vegetables and their juices

The best are sprouts. Sprouts contain up to 200 times the life force of grown foods.

Until teeth and digestion are ready, vegetables can be put through a blender. Use them in hot soups and in salads. Root vegetables should be steamed until just turning soft, then mash or put through the blender.

To make delicious and nutritious soups, select a variety of greens or other vegetables. Cut them into chunks. Put them in a blender. Add boiling water and a little sea salt. Blend for 30 seconds and serve.

Vegetable powders (dehydrated vegetables), available at health stores, make excellent soups and snacks. Mix them with hot water and add a little onion or herbal spice.

As soon as teeth chewing is possible, raw carrots, celery, raw potatoes, yams and other crisp foods exercise the jaws and help teeth grow.

Fresh fruits and their juices

Use mostly fruits that are locally grown. Those excellent for infants are the raw, scraped apples, apple sauce; also prunes or apricots, which have been soaked in spring water for 24 hours. Stewing with heat is not necessary.

Two-to-three teaspoons of freshly squeezed lemon juice in a glass of warm spring water with a teaspoon of honey is an excellent way to start the day for children (as well as adults).

Avoid full glasses of orange and grapefruit juices. They contain an excess amount of citric acid. Citrus fruits are intended by nature to supply the needs of those living in hot climates and those who perspire a great deal. People in colder climates should use citrus juices in moderation. Very active children can benefit with drinking a glass full of them.

Dried fruits: prunes, raisins, dates, figs and apricots are very good when the baby is ready for them. They are delicious when put through the blender.

Steamed Brown Rice

This can be added to any vegetable to make a purée. It blends nicely and balances food values, and stops foods from being too runny. Try steamed rice with a little cinnamon. Delicious!

Excellent snacks and treats for the one-year old or older child

- Mix steamed rice with green beans.
- Plain Arrowroot cookies.
- Oatmeal cookies or date squares, if made from natural ingredients.
- **Sherbets:** take a package of frozen fruits or berries. Add some fruit juice: orange, pineapple, coconut, piña colada or other choices. Add some almonds or coconut

chunks. Put all of them into a blender. Blend until smooth. Put back into the freezer until quite solid. This recipe makes a sherbet no commercial product will equal.

- **Ice Creams**: Not commercial varieties. A tasty, nutritious ice cream can be made from bananas. Put through a blender some of your baby's favorite frozen fruit. Add maple syrup and/or minced nuts or flavoring of your choice.
- **Natural popsicles:** freeze your baby's favorite fruit juice(s) in concentrate fruit cans. Insert popsicle sticks before freezing. Children enjoy sucking on them.

Don't use, carefully and constantly avoid...

- Stale fruits and vegetables.
- **Instant foods.** Chemicals, such as imitation fruit flavored drinks, instant soups, candies, sweets, Ovaltine and chocolate flavored drink mixes have no nutritious value.
- **Factory processed foods.** Factory processing can be like dropping a bomb onto a brand-new Mercedes-Benz.
- **Commercial** canned, bottled, packaged baby foods. Devitalized, colored and preserved foods.
- **The "white" foods.** Milk, white flour, white sugar, table salt, white (polished) rice and foods made from these: breads, rolls, buns, bagels, donuts, pastries, cookies, pies, macaroni, spaghetti, refined cereals, cream of wheat, and wheat-based desserts.
- **White or brown sugar.** They provide no nutrition. They energize by acting as a chemical whip.
- **Artificial foods.** Sweeteners and sugar substitutes. Absolutely no corn syrup, sucaryl, saccharin, monosodium glutamate or foods that contain the sweeteners: desserts, ice creams, candies, diet foods and drinks, etc.

- **Fat and fried foods.** Fat or cream substitutes, Crisco, rancid oils, the commercially treated and prepared oils, including mayonnaises and salad dressings, margarine, Mazola, canola and other bottled or canned oils marketed by supermarkets and ordinary stores.
- Canned, processed and prepared fancy meats, sandwich spreads, bologna and salami are health hazards.
- Do not peel foods, unless absolutely necessary. Clean them with a brush.
- **Frozen, concentrated fruit juices.** Squeeze and juice them fresh instead.
- Soft drinks, pop and synthetic, sweet juices.
- **Tap water.** Water that has stagnated in pipes for hours dissolves toxic minerals and/or metals from the pipes.
  - o Never use fluoride or chlorinated water. They have many serious toxic side-effects. They contribute to poor health and ugly teeth. They predispose to cancer.
- *Never use drugs*. Baby aspirins, antibiotics or any chemicals, except in an emergency. Effective natural and homeopathic alternatives exist that are harmless and just as effective.

PREPARING INFANTS FORMULAS

Cleaning foods

- **Apples and pears.** Wipe with a clean dry cloth.
- **Berries**. Pick over and wash with running water.
- **Grapes**. Pick over and do not dip or soak in bowls of water.
- **Leafy vegetables**. Put into a basin or tub with plenty of water. Add a small handful of cooking salt. Take out after half an hour. Pass under running water. Shake out the water.

Chopping

Chopping helps appetite appeal and food mastication. When teeth are good, never chop foods two much. Dental strength grows and gums benefit from the chewing of raw foods and from the exercise and activation of blood circulation, which results from the action of the jaws.

Keeping Foods Whole

Edible skins and cores are the most nutritious parts of many foods. Throwing away their skins creates a food imbalance. Valuable vitamins are lost. The skins are trace mineral foods. Trace minerals are as valuable as the sum of all vitamins and minerals found in foods.

Cooking and Undercooking with Heat

The longer the foods heat, the greater the destruction of nutrient values. Destruction of vitamins, enzymes and proteins starts at a temperature as low as 165 degrees F. Thoroughly cooked, baked or boiled foods lose a great deal of their wholeness.

Warming foods for an increased pleasure in their eating actually improves the degree of their digestion. Excess cooking is injurious to the stomach and to health. Undercooking preserves both the flavor and the food value. Always shorten the time of cooking and cook at the lowest temperature possible.

A diet composed solely or mainly of foods boiled, baked, roasted or sterilized however plentiful and rich, these foods originally were in protein and other nutrients are now a defective diet.

Cooking destroys Vitamin C in leafy vegetables and Vitamin C is essential to health.

The integrity of skin and of all organs depends on Vitamin C and its enzymes. Ascorbic acid is the universal protector against oxidation of all water soluble substances in the blood. A "hundred" health problems, even of a serious and lingering nature, proceed from insufficient assimilation of Vitamin C. Subtle injuries occurring to the gums and teeth require five times the normal intake of the vitamin.

Pressure cooking and microwave cooking both shatter, damage and denature proteins. Some decline of health must inevitably result.

Don't throw away water used for cooking. Use it for soups, broths and sauces.

Raw Foods

These should be the basis and essentials of every meal and form majority of a good healthy diet. This does not mean that man should live solely on raw vegetable foods. However, the natural nutrients in raw vegetables are the best sources for optimal healing, health protection and diseases prevention.

The healing effects of raw foods and the measure of their nutritional value are based on the energy and life forces they absorb and store from sun radiation. Excess cooking destroys nutrients, but also destroys the beneficial effects of sun's radiation on those foods.

Juices

The best method of extracting juices from fruits and/or vegetables is by the use of a macerating pulp-forming-type juicer than extracting the juices in a separate operation by squeezing and pressure. The centrifuge basket type juicers whip a great deal of air into the juices. The air oxidizes large amounts of enzymes. In order not to lose the benefits of those enzymes, the juices made in this fashion, must be drunk within minutes after extraction.

Food Value or Adding Flavor

Pleasing and stimulating flavors and varieties should be obtained through the knowledgeable use of herbs, spices, onions, garlic, oils, lemon juice, grapes, or other juices, other fruits and other sharp tasting foods. **Note:** onions play a considerable role in the Bulgarian diet. Cancer is less frequent among the Bulgarian populations.

Broths, Extracts and Sauces

These replace flavors lost by excessive cooking.

Food Quantities

Parents too easily believe that a child's voracious appetite is proof of a greater need for food as they rapidly grow. Or when their appetite decreases, too many anxious mothers pressure their children to add and eat several extra small snacks daily or meals.

Methods of Preparing Foods...

- When preparing an infant's formula, use only unpolluted spring water or non-fluorinated fresh water. Chlorinated water can be used after letting it stand for 24 hours. Chlorine evaporates in this time.
- When making a baby formula, instead of using skim cow's milk, add one part of thick cream to three parts of the water used.
- Do not boil waters used for drinking. Boiling destroys the vitality and life force. Boiled water is dead water.
- In the first months, if on a milk formula, use a quantity of water equivalent to half the amount of the milk used. Each month, slightly and gradually decrease the water content.

- If your baby is not getting as much formula as it needs, they will cry to tell you of its unsatisfied hunger and need for more food.
- The quantity of formula your baby will need will increase with the increase of the baby's appetite and needs.
- Essential proteins, minerals, vitamins, enzymes, oils and sugars normally found in mother's milk will be provided, by adding the following foods rich in them:
    o Bee pollen, Brewer's yeast, royal jelly
    o A little honey, or crude molasses
    o Potato peelings lightly simmered in water
- If confused about how to substitute commercially denatured baby foods with fresh, quality, alive foods, and if at a loss on how to prepare them, examine the labels on commercial baby food cans or bottles.
- Substitute quality alternatives for those that aren't nutritious: like honey instead of sugar, almond milk instead of cow's milk, sea salt instead of ordinary salt; quality oils instead of commercial oils, etc. or ask your naturopath.

INTRODUCING NEW FOODS – VALUABLE DON'TS

- *Never* introduce into the baby's regime more than one food or food mixture at a time.
- *Don't* insist that your infant eat unfamiliar foods. If initially they refuse the food, don't force it. Put it aside, perhaps the food is too difficult to chew, too unappetizing, or too highly seasoned. An allergy to a particular food is also and always a possibility to be considered. Try to introduce it again a week or a few weeks later.
- *Don't* make scenes when your baby has difficulties in eating or don't want to eat. No screaming, no bribes or

punishments. Remove the food. Let your baby wait until the next meal.

- **Don't** expect your baby to eat a meal, if a snack was eaten one to three hours earlier. If your baby has already had 32 ounces of formula in that day, it will not want any more food.
- **Never** introduce your baby to new foods when he/she is irritable, ill, upset or teething.
- **Don't get upset** if your infant gets upset and cries for no apparent, or for the smallest reasons, changes, irritations or imbalances. If their food is five minutes overdue; if the temperature of the room has varied by one degree or if they are left alone for five minutes too long.

Don't panic. Just tune in.

- Be reassuring. Hold your baby's hand or hum a tune.
- Be patient. It may take several weeks for your baby to learn to enjoy new tastes.
- Don't let your baby sit in their highchair for long periods of time. Their spines are not strong. Back fatigue can be upsetting.
- Introduce new foods while cuddling the baby and showing a little extra TLC at the same time.
- Offer only as small amount of new food, with the expectation that it will be eaten.
- Start your baby on juices of fruits and vegetables at an early date. Start by giving only one drop of the juice you wish to give. Each day add a few more drops. In about two months, by the time the baby is ready to take juices, it will be getting about two ounces a day.
- Wean your baby onto solid foods by starting with only a taste or just a teaspoon at a time.
- Offer the new food at the beginning of a meal, without other foods insight. While the baby is still hungry, and

before giving the bottle of formula, offer the new foods and the new forms of food – mashed or blended.

- Let your baby examine and touch the new food.
- Feed all foods – solids or formulas – at similar and not too hot temperatures. Test food temperatures by placing a drop or two onto the back of your hand.
- Help the baby learn how to swallow by putting food well back on the tongue.
- Feed with different size and shapes of spoons.
- Try different consistencies of cereals or blended foods. Some babies can readily move thick cereals and foods on their tongues, while others will gag on these and need them to be thinner.
- Provide new foods quite often so that your child becomes accustomed to changes and variety.
- Vary the preparation of foods. Involve your child in the selection and even the preparation processes.
- Momentarily distract your baby's attention from a new food with conversation. Especially do this if your child is trying to assert its own independence or attract attention to him or herself.
- Feed the baby at three or four-hour intervals. Children best know their needs. Let your child establish its own time cycle intervals. Let them determine the changes and variations of their cycle.
- Develop a routine. A baby that eats at the same time each day will more likely be hungry for meals.
- Try not to feed him/her at other times.
- When your baby has difficulty adapting to or tolerating certain foods, mix or blend small quantities of that food with a cereal, with a milk alternative or with other favorite and/or familiar food.
- Offer smaller servings. Encourage your child when he or she asks for second helpings.

- If your infant often rejects foods, screams at meals, he or she has a digestive problem. A good number of infants do. They may require enzymes and hydrochloric acid supplements for their stomach or pancreatic enzymes for their pancreas. Or, they may require the attention of the holistic physician.
- Stop all solid foods and feed the infant only with peppermint or chamomile tea to which a little honey has been added.
- If it is milk that is particularly difficult to digest, add a little Slippery Elm powder to the food. This is available at an herbalist or at health food stores.
- **Don't worry**. If your baby doesn't eat everything at every meal, you can be sure he/she will not starve or allow him/herself to starve or suffer.

SUPPLEMENTS (Vitamins, Minerals, Enzymes, etc)

Our bodies are made up of and need at least 55 vitamins, more than 100 minerals and trace minerals, 22 proteins and all of the essential oils. Generally available 'kids' vitamins contain only a fraction of them.

Those that are included in a particular formula are refined and chemically (drug company) processed and dead. They lack many elements required for complete and balanced nutrition.

The body is made to live only on alive foods that provide the totality of its requirements and these are all in balance. Only in whole, natural foods are all the health building elements found. Only concentrates derived from cells can totally regenerate or restore body cells.

Although the commercial vitamin supplements may make an infant feel better, feeling better is not always **being better**.

Foods produce their vitamins only upon ripening. They retain good vitamin levels only as long as they remain fresh. To be of value, they are to be eaten fresh and ripe. The so-called Vitamin C foods – the citrus fruits contain very little Vitamin

C. They are picked green and unripe. Potatoes, tomatoes and green peppers offer more Vitamin C than the commercial citrus fruits.

Bee pollen is one of the few perfect supplements. Pollen provides all of vitamins, minerals, trace minerals, proteins and life forces. It is rich in calcium. For the growth needs of bones and teeth, it can be given to infants, mixed in with cereals, vegetables or juices.

Adding pollen to the diet of a child is a strong and reliable guarantee of good health. Fish liver oils (halibut, cod) are still good sources of the Vitamins A and D. Once children are able to swallow them, it is preferable that they are taken in a 'perle' form. The perle capsules protect the oils from contact with air and resulting rancidity.

CHANGING FROM LIQUID TO SOLID FOOD

At about six months of age, the nervous system develops well and the senses of taste allow the child to notice if the food is appealing and appetizing. When making the change to quality food eating, start first with juices or fruits, berries, vegetables, even different kinds of nuts, such as in almond milk. This regime has curative properties for the stomach, as well as for other health problems.

"Many baby feeding problems are created by starting solid foods too early in infancy. Prematurely feeding babies solid foods, predisposes them to a lifetime of weight problems." – Dr. S. Hammar, University of Washington

Infants vary in age when their ability to swallow solid foods develop. Never feed an infant a solid food until they have enough upper and lower teeth to make good chewing possible.

Teeth appearance and the time to switch to solid foods can take place any time from four months to six months on. The decision when to accept solids always rests with your child.

At the time teeth erupts and provides good mastication, the rest of the digestive system starts to secrete the enzymes required for digesting solid foods. Before this time, a baby's throat muscles and the digestive organs are underdeveloped. Swallowing solid foods is difficult.

Any need for nutrients found only in solid foods can be offset by liquefying them, then mixing them with a nut milk or with juices and giving them in a bottle with a nipple in which the hole has been enlarged. To make a nipple hole larger, insert a heated needle into the nipple's original hole.

A BLENDER AND/OR A SEED (COFFEE) MILL: YOUR BABY'S BEST FRIEND

All milk substitutes, solid foods, grain cereals, soups, internal organ meats, fruits and vegetables are simply, and beautifully adapted to a baby's needs and to a mother's convenience by the valuable tool of a blender or coffee mill. Many foods can be blended and quickly frozen into meal-sized portions and stored; ready for quick use at any time.

Make your own baby foods by using a blender. This not only saves a lot of money, but it saves on a lot of medical bills and a parent's anguish as well. It is a time saver, energy saver and footwork saver.

ESTIMATING BABY FORMULA NEEDS

- Quantities for any of the above formula are not definite or fixed. The needs of every baby is different and vary as they grow.
- Sometimes only trial and error can best reveal the portions of servings and sizes of meals.
- If the baby does not drink all of its formula, the quantity you served is more than required.
- If the baby still cries or shows signs of hunger, the portions suggested should be increased.
- If the stools become light or grayish, add some flax seeds and sunflower oil to the formula. These activate a

better flow of bile from, and a better flushing out, of the baby liver.

- For both a better flavor and for a valuable source of energy, add a little honey to "milks" made from nuts and/or seeds. Milk, made from blended coconut, maybe sweet enough without adding too much honey.
- Enough formula can be prepared for several feedings. Store the surpluses in the refrigerator.

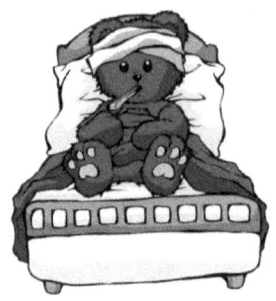

3 COMMON INFANT AILMENTS

Growing pains for infants and toddlers can be difficult, not only for the child, but the parents too. Most of the common problems, including those listed below, can usually be handled by simple and natural remedies, precautions and concentrated food supplements.

Indigestion

Most indigestion problems are from a congenital lack of stomach enzymes and hydrochloric acid. Over 10 percent of children are born with this deficiency. Proteins cannot be properly digested without this acid. The deficiency of hydrochloric acid can cause many subtle and sometimes difficult to determine health problems.

The food which most frequently triggers indigestion is milk. Over one third of children are allergic to cow's milk. This is the first thing to suspect when the child regurgitates or vomits, or rejects his bottle of milk. Adding hydrochloric acid helps relieve this. Hydrochloric plays an equally important role in the absorption and the utilization of minerals. There is no health without them. They are required in all body functions.

Increasing the intake of good quality (unpasteurized) apple cider vinegar also helps.

During the first months of life, the salivary gland does not secrete enough saliva with their sugar digesting enzymes to adequately digest starch foods, cereals, grains and the root vegetables. These foods must be kept out of the infant's diet until teeth and the saliva glands are fully functioning.

Other than the above, adding refined sugar to formula and diet is the most common cause of digestive problems and infant ill health.

Refined sugars (white or brown)...

- Interfere with the absorption of calcium and phosphorus.
- Are detrimental to the formation of bones and teeth.
- Favor the incidence of diabetes and cancer.
- Cause attacks of convulsions in some babies.

Starch breaks down into sugar when digested. Excessive quantities of cereals, root vegetables and fruits, with their high starch content, can contribute to digestive problems.

Colic

For relief of colic, make a tea by mixing catnip, fennel, peppermint or spearmint herbs. Add one teaspoon of the herbs to one cup of boiling water. Remove from heat. Cover and let steep for five to 10 minutes and strain. Add honey to taste. Each of these herbs can be effective when used singly. Other effective herbs are: caraway seed, carrot seeds, dill, Wintergreen, Valerian, Burnett, Summer Savory and Masterwort,

Measles, Chicken Pox and Mumps

Measles, Chicken Pox and Mumps are conditions resulted from:

- A combination of vitamin/mineral deficiencies
- Excess toxicities
- General low level of health and of immunity

Children's infectious diseases are usually prevented by providing all their body needs and correcting all their deficiencies.

The natural body defenses are more effective in handling these diseases than drugs, antibiotics and vaccinations. Vaccinations' complications and side effects can be more serious than the diseases they are supposed to prevent – and often don't. If a body's natural immunity and defenses are maintained by good nutrition, supported properly, it is rare that a drug or antibiotic needs to be administered.

If the child with a healthy well-nourished body still comes down with a childhood infection-type illness, their stronger health and immunity will allow only a mild attack with fairly prompt natural recuperation. There will be no after effects.

Using naturopathic approaches is recommended to build and maintain a child's immunity. Homeopathy is an option should parents decide to use it as an alternative approach to help with boosting their infant's immune system.

Feed the infant....

- Lemon juice or herbal teas with honey – lots of juices
- Calcium (lactate)
- Food-form Vitamin C complex
- Cod or halibut liver oils
- Homeopathic remedies can be specific and very effective
- Echinacea herbs or drops

Colds

Colds are 'spring cleaning' periods of body cleansing and detoxification. Bodies empty themselves of toxins, via the lungs, nose and sinuses when accumulated body garbage has overloaded the liver beyond its capacity to cope with them.

Once acquired, the cold virus attaches itself to the lining of the nasal (nose) passages and sinuses. Symptoms include a tickle in the throat, runny nose, and sneezing. Initially, discharge from the nose is clear and thin. Later it changes to a thick, yellow or greenish discharge. Young children often develop a fever of up to 102°F (39°C).

Colds can make children more susceptible to bacterial infections, such as strep throat, middle ear infection and sinus infections. The following table differentiates between the two types of infections:

Viral Infections	Bacterial Infections
Involve various parts of body:	Usually "localized" in single area:
Sore throat, runny nose, headaches, muscle ache, cough, fever, nausea and diarrhea	Sore throat, ear pain, dark phlegm, painful sinuses and urination
Cold, respiratory flu, stomach flu	Strep throat, ear infection, pneumonia
Antibiotics do not help	Antibiotics help
Rest, fluids and symptomatic relief do help	Rest, fluids and symptomatic relief
If neglected, may lead to bacterial infection	If neglected, may reduce antibiotic ineffectiveness

Other signs of a cold are coughing, sneezing, nasal congestion, headache, muscle ache, chills, sore throat, hoarseness, watery eyes, tiredness and lack of appetite. The cough that accompanies a cold is usually intermittent (it comes and goes) and dry.

Cough is a reaction that the body has when a substance irritates air passages and occurs when cells along the air passages get irritated, and trigger a chain of events. A cough is usually initiated to clear a buildup of phlegm (mucus) in the trachea. When coughing becomes very frequent or chronic, it is a sign that a disease is present in the body. Other causes of chronic cough include chronic bronchitis and medications such as ACE inhibitors. Coughing can happen voluntarily, as well as involuntarily.

Infections, such as common colds, sinus infections, pneumonia and whooping cough can result in acute coughing, whereas noninfectious causes of cough include flare-ups of the following chronic conditions: chronic bronchitis, emphysema, asthma and environmental allergies.

The overloaded elimination organ manifest as a cold can be readily controlled in several ways:

- Cleaning out the liver by the use of foods or herbs that intensify its detoxification abilities, such as a high concentrate of beet or milk thistle supplements.
- Oxidizing those toxins by taking large doses of Vitamin C.
- Fasting while taking plenty of water and herbal teas with a little honey.
- Honey and water; hip or fenugreek tea with honey.

Flues

The flu is sometimes confused with the common cold. But the flu is accompanied by more severe symptoms, including a fever. The most important indication that it is the flu rather than a cold is high fever. Flu fevers tend to be at least 102.5, 103 or 104°F and even higher in children. Since the virus attacks their whole body, they will experience weakness, tiredness, loss of appetite, severe muscle aches, headache and a cough. Allergies can also cause cold-like symptoms, but allergy symptoms last much longer than cold symptoms.

The chart below lists the differences between the common symptoms of the flu and the common cold. (ref. 6, 7)

Symptom	Flu	Cold
Fever	Usually present, high (102°F to 104°F or 38°C to 41°C); lasts 3 to 4 days	Uncommon
Headache	Very common	Uncommon
Aches and pains	Common and often severe	Slight
Fatigue and weakness	Can last up to 14-to-21 days	Mild
Extreme exhaustion	Very common at the start	Never
Stuffy nose	Sometimes	Common
Sneezing	Sometimes	Common
Sore throat	Sometimes	Common
Cough	Common and non-productive, (non-mucous producing) dry cough	Mild to moderate, hacking cough
Causative organism	Adenoviruses, coronaviruses or rhinoviruses	Influenza virus

The best defense in beating the cold and flu season is to boost you and your child's immune system.

Natural supplements like Vitamin C and Echinacea can also be used to help boost the immune system. Natural sources of Vitamin C are citrus fruits, cantaloupe, berries, green peppers, leafy green vegetables, cauliflower, potatoes, tomatoes, broccoli, oranges, peppers, grapefruit, papaya and strawberries.

- Vitamin C is a requirement for the proper functioning of our immune systems.
- It is involved in white blood cell production, T-cells and macrophages.
- Ascorbic acid is toxic to viruses, bacteria and many types of cultured cells, because of its anti-oxidant activity.
- It is particularly toxic to malignant tumor cells, but much less toxic to nonmalignant normal cells.
- Although the RDI is less than 100mg, it is recommended to take 500mg two-to-four times a day as a treatment for colds.

Echinacea has been popularly attributed with the ability to boost the body's immune system and ward off infections, particularly the common cold. Depending on which species is used, herbal medicinal can be prepared from the above-ground parts and/or the root. The main species are *P. purpurea*, *E. angustifolia*, and *E. pallida*. Echinacea is sometimes used as a natural antibiotic and immune system stimulator, helping to build resistance to colds, flu and infections. It is thought to stimulate the production of white blood cells, and improve the lymph glands. The constituents of Echinacea include essential oil, polysaccharides, polyacetylenes, betain, glycoside, sesquiterpenes and caryophylene. It also contains copper, iron, tannins, protein, fatty acids and Vitamins A, C, and E.

Echinacea has traditionally been used to treat or prevent colds, flu, and other infections.
Echinacea is believed to stimulate the immune system to help fight infections.
Less commonly, Echinacea has been used for wounds and skin problems, such as acne.

Our bodies have immune agents that fight against viruses. Those specific to viruses are body combinations of special oils and phosphorus called phospholipids.
The main and richest source of phospholipids is unrefined, unprocessed concentrated soy lecithin.

Botanical Medicines

Botanical medicines have many advantages and a great complement to other forms of medicine. They have extraordinary versatility. For example, if one has a cold then the practitioner would first deal with the infection using antibiotics and then give a drug for the cough. However, in herbal medicine, a complementary approach would be to use different herbs, dependent upon the type of cough. For an irritant cough, demulcents or soothing expectorants, which coat and soothe the irritated tissues, would be used. Stimulating expectorants could be used in cases of chronic congestion, such as chronic bronchitis.

Chamomile

- Anti-inflammatory, antispasmodic, anti-infective, calmative, mild sedative.
- Reduces anxiety. Good anti-bacterial action.
- Reduces inflammations of the mucous membrane.
- Calms nerves. Calms upset stomach.

Calendula

Anti-inflammatory, granulator and wound healing action with topical application, inflammation of the oral and pharyngeal mucosa. It was also approved externally for poorly healing wounds. Specially, herbal infusions, tincture and ointments are used to respond to skin and mucous membrane inflammations, such as pharyngitis, dermatitis, leg ulcers, bruises, boils and rashes.

Dandelion

Anti-rheumatic, diuretic, tonic.
Aids healing of kidney and liver disorders, natural diuretic, digestive aid, reduces blood pressure. Appears to help prevent iron-deficiency, anemia, chronic rheumatism, gout and stiff joints.

Lavender

Sedative for restlessness, sleeplessness, lack of appetite.
Nervous, irritable stomach.
Meteorism and nervous disorders of the intestines.

Rosehips
Astringent, diuretic, tonic
Great source of Vitamin C for stressful and nervous situations.
Blood purifier, used for infections.

Valerian

Antispasmodic, anodyne, carminative, hypnotic, nervine, hypotensive, sedative, stimulant.
Beneficial for insomnia, nervousness, anxiety, panic attacks and times of extreme emotional stressful feelings. Alleviates gas, pains, spasms and other general conditions due to stress, such as muscle cramps due to PMS and menstrual cramps.

Antioxidants

- Antioxidant is a catchall term for any compound that can counteract unstable molecules, such as free radicals that damage DNA, cell membranes and other parts of cells.
- Antioxidants are those amino acids, enzymes, minerals, vitamins and supplements that prevent or control the oxidative process, which is like rusting the body from inside and outside.
- Antioxidants are the scavengers which protect your body from free radical damage. Free radicals are the negative byproduct created when the body produces energy or due to the body's reaction to such things as air pollution, sunshine, diseases, illnesses, food carcinogens like nitrates, curing and smoke from charcoal barbecues, emotional or mental stress and almost all activities of daily life to one degree or another. They are responsible for the damaging process which is caused by uncontrolled oxidation and damages cells, as well as weaken the immune system.

They lack a full complement of electrons, which makes them unstable, so they steal electrons from other molecules, damaging those molecules in the process.

One example of this harm is when free radicals attack low-density lipoproteins (LDL,

the "bad" cholesterol) that have made their way into the cells lining artery walls. After giving up their electrons, the LDL molecules become more reactive compounds that can injure the arterial lining and spark a cascade of events that, with repeated occurrences, can eventually narrow the artery.

- Antioxidants that occur naturally in the body and certain foods may block this damage by donating electrons to stabilize and neutralize the harmful effects of the free radicals.

- **Carotenoids** - lycopene in tomatoes and lutein in kale, beta-carotene in carrots, Co Q 10.

- **Flavonoids**, such as anthocyanins in blueberries.

- **Quercetin** in apples and onions.

- **Catechins** in green tea.

- **Isoflavones**, such as those found in soy products like genistein and daidzein.

Fruits: prunes or dried plums, blueberries and cherries, purple berries (elderberry, black currant) and cranberries.
Vegetables: artichokes, red cabbage and russet potatoes. Beans and Brussels sprouts were also touted to have a large amount of antioxidant capacity.
Nut: pecans, walnuts and hazelnuts.
Spices: Oregano, cinnamon, and cloves are included in the antioxidant food list.

Inflammation of the nose, ears, throat, lungs or sinuses

Sugars, pasteurized milk, refined wheat foods, overcooked proteins foods and junk foods, contribute to inflammation of the mucous membrane linings of the nose, ears, sinuses, lungs and to build up mucus, stuffy nose and sinus congestion.
All infections, conditions are greatly helped by Vitamin A and C and calcium (preferably lactate) with magnesium. In combination, these act as effectively as a mild antibiotic.

Echinacea and homeopathic remedies are equally effective.

Overfeeding

This also can cause inflammations and infections. Whatever excesses go into the body, must come out. If not eliminated, they overload the organs of detoxification and elimination (liver, kidneys and lungs), and add to the inflammations, colds, coughs, lung congestion and pneumonia. Excesses of the mucus-producing foods (again milk, wheat, sugar, refined and processed and unnatural foods) can cause pneumonia.

Milk intolerances are always suspect to a faulty digestion or an allergy.

Intolerances manifest by…

- Changes of color, consistency and solidity of stools.
- Colic, cramps, long periods of crying.
- Regurgitating or vomiting.
- Constipation or diarrhea.

Teething

Foods and factors that reduce gum sensitivity so that teeth can come through with a minimum of discomfort are:

- Generous intakes of calcium/magnesium supplements.
- Generous intakes of calcium rich foods: the crisp, brittle foods, unpasteurized cheese, but never pasteurized milk.
- Body saturation of the minerals and oils

Rubbing cloves into the tender gums is an excellent way of reducing gum and cavity tenderness, and pain. Gentle rubbing or massaging the gums with chamomile drops can also help soothe the pain. Fevers that accompany teething can be controlled by intakes of calcium, together with Vitamin C and Vitamin A complexes (with their enzymes and synergists). These counsels have given real relief to many children.

Insomnia, restless sleep and unpleasant dreams

Quiet relaxing sleep is most essential to health. During sleep is when body healing and restoration takes place.
A body that is too acid is energized, tense and active. Excess diet acidity interferes with sleep and rest, and with the healing. Alkalizing foods (and supplements) slow down body activity and relax the nervous system in ways that are conducive to normal, quiet and relaxing sleep. Excellent relaxing herbal teas are available at health stores.

Alfalfa-type supplements are rich sources of potassium, the most alkaline mineral.

The only alkalizing foods are vegetables and fruits (except cranberries, prunes and plums) and their juices. Honey is a very relaxing food. It can often successfully induce sleep in infants when even sedatives won't.

Fatigue, Sluggishness

Depletion of alkaline mineral reserves is a reduction in body energies, vitality and health reserves. Major roles of the alkaline minerals are to create body strength and endurance. They provide the glands with the elements that they need to create the hormones which are body, mind and muscle activators and accelerators.

Skin and Buttocks Rashes and Irritants

Skin rashes invariably are caused by...

- Excess levels of body toxins (toxic causes above).
- Excess body acidity – mostly from excess acid foods.

- Excess body alkalinity – low hydrochloric acid.
- A deficiency of quality oils (whose role it is to form a coating around cell membranes, like a shield or suit of armor) is a failure of the skin to protect itself from the onslaught of toxins, acids and alkaline.
- Oils protect skin cells from being damaged by toxic secretion coming from the skin.

Cradle Cap

Cradle cap is a greasy crust on the scalp. Soften at night with lanolin. In the morning, wash thoroughly with chickweed tea or apply a thin solution of baking soda and water to the scalp. Leave it on overnight. Shampoo in the morning and use sage as an excellent rinse.

Diaper Rash

Giving baby lots of water is often all that is required to prevent diaper rash. If it is not effective, soothe the rash with a tea made from potato skins, grated cucumber or from two teaspoons of chickweed to a cup of warm water (not chlorinated, fluorinated or direct from the tap). Let dry. If possible, do this in the sunlight. Vitamin E ointment is excellent. "The best form of Vitamin E is wheat germ oil." (Dr. Evan Shute, the discoverer of Vitamin E).
Slightly brown (roasted in oven), white flour makes an excellent powder to keep the baby's bottom dry. Calendula cream can also be used for many dermatological conditions.

Constipation: Its Causes

There must always be as many bowel movements per day as there are substantial meals. A less number generally results from… faulty digestion of foods, resulting from an inadequate secretion of digestion enzymes.

Inadequately digested foods rot, ferment or putrefy. These resulting toxic substances intoxicate, drug, slow down or paralyzes the bowel wall muscle, which expels fecal matter, making their contractions and expansions sluggish.

Diarrhea

Treat with...

- Probiotics
- Digestive enzymes
- Teething remedies, as described on previous pages
- Increased fiber-rich foods: bran, salads, carrots, nuts and raw foods (avoid the All Bran cereal).

Diminished acuteness of vision (shortsightedness): especially during periods of intensive growth.

Digestive troubles: loss or decrease of appetite. Remember that the organs that perform the processes of digestion (no less than other organs), also need times for rest and regeneration.

Acne: psoriasis, urticaria, eczema and other skin troubles...
Almost without exception, these are the results of the wrong diet. They yield only to a fundamental change of dietetic errors.

Anemia (blood problems): The composition of the blood depends upon diet and the collaboration of all body organs. The blood develops healthy capillaries and of the whole body. Meaty diets with their excess acidity, over a period of only 10 days, cause the bloodstream to become congested and blood flow becomes retarded. The flow of nutrients to organs and to the cells deteriorate.

Capillary problems

The capillaries make up a total length of 1500 miles of

surface. This is the equivalent of 100 square yards in each body. This promotes the body's internal food absorption and waste disposal. The development of the capillary network occurs only in the second or fourth year in infants.

Capillaries determine the effectiveness, the capacity and the speed flow of the nutrients through the blood. Health and life depends on them.

Capillaries development is retarded by nutrient deficiencies and imbalances. The causes of any faulty development are similar to those causing goiter and cretinism. The results: immaturity and mental retardation.

Capillary Damaged by Malnutrition

In the development of capillary loops – hairpin shaped loops – become distorted through abnormal diet. They can contract and shrivel. This interferes with food absorption and toxin elimination.

Ulcers and Colitis

In experiments, Dr. McCarrison gave steamed, pressure cooked foods to apes. Within 100 days, all of them developed colitis and ulcers. Other results of the same steamed, pressured cooked foods are degeneration of the salivary glands, anemia, scurvy, rheumatoid arthritis, goiter and cancer.

Cyanosis (abnormal redness of color), paleness and heart disease are related to the blood and capillaries.

Diet influences growth with peculiar intensity

"It is progressively becoming more accepted that man is composed of what he eats. Defects in the architecture of the human body are largely due to defects in the quality of food, especially during the growing period of life. These defects are often at the root of disease processes, which manifest themselves clinically in later life. But these can be prevented. Even when defects have produced cell changes, these (if not too far advanced or complicated by superimposed infection) can be rectified by correcting defects in the composition and balance of the diet." - Dr. McCarrison, *British Medical Journal*

Rickets

This is caused by the lack of Vitamin D and a wrong proportion of phosphorus and calcium in food and the blood. Vitamin D, in an active state, exists in unrefined cod and halibut liver oils, and to a lesser degree, in egg yolks.
The sun's rays are an important and vital factor in the nutrition of mankind and particularly of children. Ergosterol and similar substances, contained in certain foods, are taken into our bodies as preliminary stages of vitamin D formation.
They are stored in the skin. Sunlight, which penetrates the skin, activates the substances. Vitamin D is produced from ergosterol. It influences growth and hardening of growing bones and teeth by promoting the absorption and storing up of calcium in these tissues.

Almost every child in mid-European countries is affected even if only slightly, by its consequences. These are: warping, crookedness and deformities of the long bones; knock knees, bandy legs, curvatures of the spine, flatness of the chest, asymmetrical skull, abnormal positioning of teeth, diminished power of mastication, faculty teeth clenching, and narrow pelvis. These often appear during years of intensive growth, from fifth to seventh year, and from 12th to 16th years.

Secondary consequences of rickets

- Decreased well-being of general health.
- Decreased state of the nervous system.
- Increased susceptibility to fatigue.
- Tendency to idleness.

- Heightened reflexes.
- Hyper-excitability, nervous character.

Loss of natural immunity against infections

A defective diet increases susceptibility to colds, catarrh and tonsillitis and even to tuberculosis. Natural immunity can be achieved only by means of proper diet.

Acid Alkaline Imbalances

Too much acidity and excess intake of strongly acid food substances – proteins, fats, carbohydrates and sugars – impair general health and body structures of the growing human being.

Effects of excess acidity

- Weakening of the muscular system.
- A weakened constitution.
- Increased growth in the length of the long bones.
- Long thin, narrow, pigeon shaped, or pear-shaped chest.
- Underdeveloped or infantile uterus.
- Susceptibility to juvenile diseases.
- Excess tallness, precociousness and increased height are indications of general body health deterioration.
- Precociousness usually goes with excess growth.

Hyperactivity effects

- Inability to concentrate.
- Nervousness, irritability.
- Poor sleep.
- Personality changes and problems.

Hyperactivity of Children

This state is the effect on the body of...

- High acid foods, highly toxic foods, high body pH.
- Diets with soft drinks, caffeine, coffee, chocolate.
- Sugars, candies, ice cream and desserts.
- Diets high in fat foods, but low in quality oils.
- The chemicals in foods and in one's environment.
- Pasteurized/homogenized milk.
- Prepared and canned/bottled baby foods.
- Ordinary table salt.
- Losses of calcium.
- Poor intake of the quality crisp, calcium rich foods.
- Overstimulation of a hypersensitive nervous system.
- Excess exposure to fluorescent lights.
- Tensions, fears, angers, stress in those around the child.
- Criticism, dissatisfaction, excess punishments.
- Accumulations of body waste products as these stagnate in the blood and tissues.
- Insufficient enzymes to metabolize. Excess tenseness, over activity and crying infants generally indicates colic from indigestion. If minerals are not digested, absorbed and utilized, the body condition turns excessively acid. In other words: low stomach acid = little mineral reserve = high body acidity.

Excess acids can be found in sweets, desserts, candies and fancy cereals. Many vitamin pills are strongly acidic. One bottle of a soft drink contains acid levels so high that if all its acids were absorbed into a body, it could take up to one month to break them down and use them.

Excess acids, which are not the body's normal acids, (vinegar, soft drinks, sugar, sweets and wheat diets), will keep too many alkaline minerals in a dissolved state. With a body's discharge of fluids, they are flushed through the kidneys. This loss of minerals also results in an excessively acid body state.

Warm, fresh squeezed lemon juice with honey is a good body alkalizer and relaxant. It is a good way to start the day for tense, easily upset children (parents as well).

Ear Aches and Complaints

Ear aches, deafness and ear infections are usually brought on by excesses of mucus forming foods: milk, wheat, sugar, overcooked proteins and non-nutrient foods.

Mild to moderate earache can be a sharp, dull or burning pain, which can occur in one or both ears. (Ref.1)

Chronic otalgia (earache) is a common occurrence usually for many adults, but can happen in children as well. The ear pain felt may be coming from the teeth, stress, joints in the jaw or throat, trauma and loud noises. (Ref. 2)

- Initially, one has to look at elimination of foods that may be contributing to poor immunity, as well as allergies to help with chronic ear pain.
- Warm compress near the ear that is clogged and throbbing reduces pain and discomfort very quickly.
- Over-the-counter ear drops can be used to relieve pain, as long as the eardrum has not ruptured.
- Juices from garlic help relieve the symptoms associated with upper respiratory tract infections and catarrhal conditions. (Ref. 3)

Vitamin C taken internally is a very good supplement, which is an antioxidant for the maintenance of good health. (Ref. 4)

Zinc helps to maintain immune function. (Ref. 5)

Echinacea is used to help fight off infections, especially of the upper respiratory tract. (Ref. 6)

Besides acupuncture, homeopathy can also be considered. Belladonna is the most commonly indicated homeopathic medicine during the early stages of an ear infection or earache. Others to consider include Hepar, sulph, Pulsatilla and Chamomilla. (Ref. 7)

Prevention

The following steps can help prevent earaches:

- Avoid smoking.
- Chewing or sucking may help relieve the pain and pressure of an ear infection.
- Prevent outer ear infections by not putting objects in the ear.
- Resting in an upright position instead of lying down can reduce pressure in the middle ear.
- Dry the ears well after bathing or swimming.

MAJOR CAUSES OF INFANT ILLNESS

All toxins, as listed throughout this book.

- All the abnormal and junk nutrients previously described.
- Toxins from abnormal digestion.
- Allergies and intake of allergens.
- Chemicals, drugs.
- Preservatives, additives, artificial food colors.
- Synthetic fabrics of baby's clothes and diapers.
- Chemical soaps and chemicals skin lotions.
- Food, water and air pollutants.

Bile Deficiency

Bile activates the intestinal muscles and retains the oils which serve as an intestinal lubricant. Pale bowel movements tell us that bile resources are low.

Normalize the stools and its color...

- Take bile tablets.
- Eliminate the denatured oils and fats in the diet.
- Moderate the use of nuts, almonds and their milks.
- Switch from nut milks to soya milk unless stools are a normal dark brown color.
- Strengthen the liver functions by the use of liver cell extract concentrates.

Drugs, Antibiotics

Antibiotics are useless and powerless for about 90 percent of the illnesses from which the children suffer. They have no ability to control viruses. Avoiding the causes of diseases is the best way to avoid the needs for antibiotics.

Antibiotics destroy the normal intestinal bacteria and their function of breaking down fecal matter, body wastes, and poisons, preparing them for elimination.

Lack of adequate "friendly bacteria" can result from too much antibiotic treatment, constipation and a diet that is low in calcium, fiber, lactose and other complex carbohydrates. Since diet has a major influence on the profile of the intestinal flora, antagonists to friendly bacterial proliferation will result in an overgrowth of coliforms and other "unfriendly" bacteria.

Just like the body needs fiber to function optimally, it needs good bacteria. Friendly bacteria are responsible for defending the body against disease and infection, and prevent overtaxing its immune system.

Good bacteria: Fighting the Good Fight!

Good bacteria aid in preventing fungal and yeast infections from overwhelming the body, and instrumental in producing B vitamins. It also helps the digestive system, plus a host of other activities beneficial to a child's health and wellbeing.

If your child needs to use pharmaceutical antibiotics, their body's natural bacteria balance will be disturbed. Unfortunately, synthetic antibiotics destroy all the bacteria, good and bad, in their path. They may offer temporary relief from gastrointestinal problems, but at a price beyond relief. The child's immune system (and yours) become weakened and more susceptible to diseases and infections until his or her body rebuilds it natural defense mechanism. Bad bacteria become resistant to antibiotics, which is part of the reason we are having outbreaks of "super resistant bad bacteria" which can be life threatening. The answer is to restore the good bacteria levels in your child's gut, as gently and as soon as possible.

Studies have shown that probiotics are an answer to some gastrointestinal issues in children. Probiotics come in a variety of forms that they may enjoy taking: drops or chewable tablets, as well as supplements. Don't forget creating healthy meals that include yogurt with the good bacterial culture (preferably organic).

Dietary fiber is also a feeding ground for bacteria. They metabolize the fiber, turning it into acids which reduce the growth rates of bad bacteria. Berries, pears, almonds are an example of good fiber that children will love consuming.

It is highly recommended to supplement with a probiotic when your child starts taking an antibiotic, and for at least 30 days when they have finished the prescription. Give them the probiotic a half hour before each meal. They may experience some gas or bloating. It indicates that their system is adjusting to the probiotic. Fermentation is the process that is occurring in their gut. The problem should clear itself up, once their body adjusts, usually within 10 days.

"Doctors use too many antibiotics in treating children with coughs, sore throats and runny nose." - Dr. Donald Stewart, Medical Director of the Outpatients Department of Toronto's Hospital for Sick Children.

FOOD CAUSES OF BABY ILLNESSES

The *wrong types of food* in the diet.

Pasteurized milk: *one* glass a day can decrease bowel elimination by a one movement a day.

White flour in the diet: mixing white flour and water (or other liquid) in the intestines, makes glue – the same as making paste from the same mixture in a bowl. The fecal matter becomes thick, sluggish and slow to remove.

Sugars: these are too acidic. They deplete the calcium and minerals, the muscles of the intestines require in order to contract and expand, bringing about the flushing of fecal matter.

Overcooked foods: never cooked foods until they are soft and mushy.

Caffeine: damages chromosomes. In particular, the caffeine content in chocolate is higher than coffee. Coffee, black tea, cocoa and chocolate are to be eliminated. The addition of refined sugar to these is more objectionable. They markedly excite the nervous system and the most delicate blood vessels. They fill the body, leaving less space or appetite instinct for providing the body with its essential needs. The sugar content in chocolate is excessive. Bodies injured by chocolate are difficult to heal.

Viruses and Bacteria

These are the result of illnesses children have – not their cause. Microbes grow on and are fostered by body poisons – the real causes of infectious diseases.

Medications can cause skin rashes, fevers, swollen glands, dehydration and gastro-enteritis. Often these symptoms are misinterpreted as being diseases. The newly diagnosed "disease" may be treated with more drugs. These, in turn, may cause more side effects.

Furthermore, the promiscuous use of antibiotics promotes the development of "super germs" – germs like meningitis and staphylococcus. Eventually, overuse of antibiotics can lead to resistance to penicillin and other anti-infection drugs.

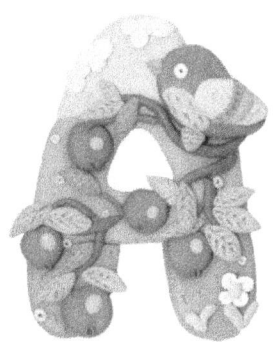

4 ALLERGIES & ASTHMA
TODAY'S PREVALENT AILMENTS

I'm giving a separate chapter to allergies and asthma, because both are so prevalent in today's world. At least 90 percent of the population suffers from an allergy and over 11.6 million children in North America have asthma.

Please keep in mind that most of the naturopathic solutions provided in this chapter, pertain primarily to the adult. However, it has been determined that some of the solutions can also be administered to children in lesser dosages. How do you determine the dosage for your child? You can use either the Clark's Rule or the Young's Rule. They are methods by which you can calculate pediatric dosages according to a child's weight and size, because the manufacturer has not provided recommended dosages for children or your holistic practitioner would like to use the medicine.

Clark's Formula: * Uses Weight in Lbs, *NEVER* in Kg.

Adult Dose X (Weight ÷ 150) = Childs Dose

For Example:
A 11 year old girl at 70 Lbs

500mg X (70 ÷ 150) = Child's Dose

500mg X (.47)= Child's Dose

500mg X .47 = 235mg

Child's Dose = 235Mg

The Young's Formula: * Uses Age

Adult Dose X (Age ÷ (Age+12)) = Child's Dose

For Example
11 year old girl's weight is 70 Lbs

500mg X (11 ÷ (11+12)) = Child's Dose

500mg X (11 ÷ 23) = Child's Dose

500mg X .48 = Child's Dose

Child's Dose = 240mg

It is highly recommended that if you are unclear about the dosage, visit with your child's pediatrician or holistic practitioner.

FOOD INTOLERANCES

About 95 percent of infants born in recent years will have some form of an allergy. Fifty years ago, possibly no more than five percent of infants had allergies. Sometimes allergies manifest in noticeable ways only as the child grows up.

An allergy is sometimes a mild, sometimes latent, sometimes strong physical, mental or emotional reaction, arising from a hypersensitivity to a substance which is normally harmless and from a failure of the body's ability to chemically process or handle (metabolize) that substance. A substance that cannot be made to fit into a child's biochemistry and into the structures and functions of his or her cells is considered a foreign substance. Not liked or compatible, it is an irritant.

As mentioned in previous chapters, the most common allergy is to milk. To avoid the trigger allergen is to constantly take a natural form of antihistamine or supplement your baby's digestion with stomach or pancreatic enzymes. This may be the only means of helping or controlling allergies.

Quality cow's milk causes other ailments, such as bedwetting, proneness to heart attacks, neutralization of stomach acids and impaired digestion later on in life.

Good tolerance and digestion of fats, as well as indications of the amounts of fats and oils that can be normally used by the baby, will be indicated by its bowel movement: solidity, freedom from gas, fibers or undigested foods and normal, dark brown color. If the bowel movements become slightly pale, or if there is constipation, there is also liver fatigue or congestion. The liver is not secreting enough bile.

HAY FEVER

Hay fever is inflammation of the nasal passages. It is an allergic reaction to substances present in the air. The medical name for hay fever is *allergic rhinitis*. Allergies tend to run in families and it's believed that breastfed babies are less likely to develop allergies as they grow up.

Hay fever is the most common allergic condition. An allergic condition is a reaction by the body to some substance that is harmless to most people. For example, most people are not bothered by dust in the air. For others, however, inhaling dust can cause dramatic bodily changes, such as sneezing, coughing and itchy, and watery eyes.

There are two types of hay fever (allergic rhinitis): seasonal and perennial. Seasonal hay fever occurs in the spring, summer, and early fall. During these seasons, the level of plant pollens in the air is at its highest. Perennial hay fever occurs all year. It is usually caused by substances found in the air at home or in the workplace. A person may have one or both types of hay fever. Symptoms of seasonal hay fever are worst after being outdoors. Symptoms of perennial hay fever are worst after spending time indoors. Both forms of hay fever can develop at any age. In most cases, they first appear during childhood. They may become either worse or better over time.

Hay fever is a kind of immune reaction. The immune system is an intricate defense network of white blood cells whose job it is to fight off "foreign invaders", such as bacteria and viruses. When a foreign substance enters the body, the immune system releases antibodies. Antibodies are chemicals with the ability to destroy the foreign substances.

In the case of hay fever, the immune system becomes confused. It treats dust, mold, pollen, and other harmless substances as if they are dangerous. Substances that cause this kind of reaction are known as allergens. The combination of antibody and allergen sets off a series of reactions designed to protect the body. These reactions cause cells and blood vessels to leak fluids. These fluids cause the symptoms of hay fever, such as a runny nose, red and irritated eyes, an itchy nose and a scratchy throat.

Researchers aren't sure which part of the system goes haywire in an allergic reaction. However, the immune system wrongly identifies a non-toxic substance as an invader and rallies an allergic response to protect your child. Soon, the allergic reaction, meant to protect, becomes the disease in itself.

Allergen:

A substance that provokes an allergic response.

Anaphylaxis:

Increased sensitivity caused by previous exposure to an allergen that can result in blood vessel dilation (swelling) and smooth muscle contraction. Anaphylaxis can result in sharp blood pressure drops and difficulty breathing.

Antibody:

A specific protein produced by the immune system in response to a specific foreign protein or particle called an antigen.

Granules:

Small packets of reactive chemicals stored within cells.

Histamine:

A chemical released by mast cells that activates pain receptors and causes cells to leak fluids.

Mast Cells:

A type of immune system cell that is found in the lining of the nasal passages and eyelids. It displays a type of antibody called immunoglobulin type E (IgE) on its cell surface and participates in the allergic response by releasing histamine from intracellular granules.

The number of possible allergens found in the air is enormous. Seasonal hay fever is most commonly caused by grass and tree pollen. Pollen is a fine powder by which plants are germinated. A number of weeds can also cause hay fever. These include:

- Ragweed
- Sagebrush
- Lamb's quarters
- Plantain
- Pigweed
- Dock (sorrel)
- Tumbleweed

Perennial hay fever is also caused by a variety of particles found in the air including:

- **Body parts of house mites.** House mites are tiny insects. They can be seen only with the aid of a microscope. They feed on fibers, fur, and skin shed by people who live in the house. When they die, their body parts get into the air.
- **Animal wastes.** Animals constantly shed fur, skin flakes, and dried saliva. Common sources of these materials are pet dogs, cats, and birds. These materials easily get into the air. They cause allergic reactions in many people.

- **Mold spores.** Mold is a fungus that grows in warm, damp places. It lives in basements, bathrooms, air ducts, air conditioners, refrigerator drains, mattresses, and stuffed furniture. Mold reproduces by giving off tiny seed-like particles called spores. These spores are released into the air. They can cause hay fever in many people.

Other possible causes of perennial hay fever include the following:

- Cigarette smoke
- Perfume
- Cosmetics
- Cleansers
- Chemicals used in copy machines
- Industrial chemicals
- Gases given off by construction materials, such as insulation

HAY FEVER SYMPTOMS

Common symptoms of hay fever include a tender, itchy, runny nose, accompanied by sneezing and coughing. The sinuses may also begin to swell, causing the eustachian (pronounced you-STAY-shee-un) tube to close up. The eustachian tube connects the inner ear to the throat. The closing of the eustachian tube causes a feeling of stuffiness. Mucus may drip from the sinuses into the throat, causing the throat to become sore. There is no fever associated with hay fever, but red, itchy, watery eyes (mentioned early) and fatigue, and headaches.

DIAGNOSIS

Hay fever can usually be diagnosed quite easily. Symptoms and a medical history usually indicate the presence of the condition. When symptoms appear in the spring and disappear in the fall, seasonal hay fever is likely to be the cause. Perennial hay fever can often be diagnosed by asking the patient what substances seem to cause his or her symptoms.

Skin tests are often used in diagnosing hay fever. The first step in conducting a skin test is to place a small amount of a suspected allergen on the skin. The doctor then scratches the skin very lightly. The scratch allows the allergen to get into the bloodstream. After a few minutes, the doctor checks the area being tested. A redness and swelling indicate that the patient is allergic to the material being tested. In most cases, twenty or more materials can be tested at one time. The tests are carried out on the patient's back or forearm.

Some types of drugs used to treat hay fever include the following:

- **Antihistamines.** Antihistamines block the action of histamine (pronounced HISS-tuh-meen) in the immune system. Histamine is a chemical that causes many of the symptoms of hay fever. Antihistamines can be used after the symptoms of hay fever appear, but they are more effective if used before the symptoms appear. Many older types of antihistamines caused drowsiness. Some newer types do not have this side effect.
- **Decongestants.** Decongestants constrict (shrink) blood vessels. They reduce the loss of fluid from blood vessels that causes many symptoms of hay fever. Commercial decongestants are sold in liquid forms for children. It's not recommended, however to use them for long periods of time. One dangerous side effect is that they increase

blood pressure and heart rate. They should not be taken for more than a few days at a time.

- **Topical corticosteroids.** Topical corticosteroids (pronounced kor-tih-ko-STIHR-oids) reduce inflammation and swelling of tissue. They tend to work more slowly and last longer than other forms of medication. As a result, they should be started before the hay fever season begins. It should be used in low potency versions for children to minimize any side effects.
- **Mast cell stabilizers.** Mast cells are cells produced by the immune system. They are responsible for the early stages of an allergic reaction. Mast cell stabilizers stop the allergic reaction before it gets started. They can also be used before the hay fever season begins. In that case, they reduce the chance that hay fever will develop. Your pediatrician will help you determine the right dose for your child, taking into consideration his or her age.

Some alternative practitioners believe that hay fever should be treated by strengthening the immune system. They may recommend a more balanced diet and changes in one's lifestyle.

Vitamin C is sometimes recommended to reduce inflammation of tissues. Some herbs that are recommended for relief of hay fever symptoms include eyebright, bee pollen, and nettle.

PREVENTION

There are many things a person can do to avoid allergic reactions. Some of the most common recommendations for preventing seasonal hay fever include:

- Staying indoors with windows closed during the morning hours, when pollen levels are highest.

- Keeping car windows closed while driving.
- Wearing a surgical mask when it is necessary to be outdoors.
- Avoiding trees, bushes, flowers, and other plants to which your child is allergic.
- Wash clothes and hair after being outside.
- Clean air conditioner filters in the home regularly.
- In severe cases, consider moving to an area with fewer allergens.

To reduce the symptoms of perennial hay fever, keep children away from mold spores, house dust, and animal wastes by taking steps, such as:

- Keeping the house dry through ventilation and use a dehumidifier.
- Keeping bathroom floors and walls clean with a disinfectant.
- Cleaning and disinfecting air conditioners and coolers
- Throwing out moldy or mildewed books, shoes, pillows, and furniture.
- Vacuuming frequently and change the vacuum bag regularly.
- Cleaning floors and walls with a damp mop.
- Reconsidering having a pet and/or avoid contact with pets, if the child is allergic.
- Washing hands after contact with pets and other animals.
- Keeping pets out of the bedroom, off furniture and other areas where their waste materials may collect.
- Having pets bathed and groomed regularly.

It's currently estimated that over forty million, or 25 percent of Americans, suffer from asthma, hay fever and other allergies. While over-the-counter remedies can relieve symptoms such as runny eyes and sneezing, they often leave sufferers feeling dizzy or sleepy, and are not recommended for prolonged use. These remedies do nothing to aid the body in recovery.

HERBS

Herbs, such as *eyebright, nettle* and *elder,* in dosages suitable for children, according to their weight and age (Clark's and Young's Rules), can help relieve symptoms, as well as help their bodies reach a state of balance.

Ephedra Sinica

Please note: This herb is <u>not</u> recommended for children under 18 years of age. I decided to include it if you have adult children or if you know of anyone who is suffering with allergies.

The Chinese have used *Ephedra* or the dried stems of the *Ephedra* plant, Ma huang, for at least 5000 years to treat hay fever, colds and other inflammatory conditions. From a Traditional Chinese Medicine perspective, Ma huang "facilitates the movement of lung qi and controls wheezing." It's considered to be hot, bitter and warming, and its functions are to induce sweat, soothe breath and promote the excretion of urine.

Indeed, *Ephedra* contains a number of active compounds, including small amounts of an essential oil, and most importantly, one to two percent alkaloids composed mainly of ephedrine and pseudoephedrine. Modern medicine discovered *Ephedra's* alkaloid compound ephedrine in 1923, and synthetic manufacture of ephedrine began shortly thereafter. Researchers found that ephedrine had an effect on the body very similar to that of adrenalin (used at that time to treat asthma attacks), without many of the side-effects of adrenalin (the proprietary name for the hormone epinephrine).

However, it soon became clear that ephedrine, the isolated constituent of *Ephedra,* also had unacceptable side-effects, such as elevated blood pressure that limited its use. Herbalists point out that the whole herb *Ephedra* contains numerous other components besides ephedrine that possess significant anti-inflammatory and anti-allergy activities including quercitin, which is known for its anti-inflammatory, anti-allergic and bronchiodilating qualities. The whole herb *Ephedra* also contains another alkaloid called pseudoephedrine, which is an effective bronchiodilator yet slightly reduces heart rate and blood pressure.

Some states have recently passed new laws and/or issued regulations controlling the sale of Ephedra products due to concerns about safe dosages, especially the use of phedrine-containing stimulant pills, which have become popular among high school children. Safe dosage is the key to using Ephedra. The research shows that it can dramatically reduce symptoms of watery, itchy eyes, runny nose and sneezing.

The sinuses are often involved in allergy reactions. The tissues lining these air-filled cavities above, below and behind the eyes can swell, which can block the outlets of the sinuses to the nose. Mucus buildup in the sinuses can cause headaches, while mucus draining from the back of the nose into the throat can irritate the throat. *Ephedra* is a proven, effective decongestant because its active constituents, ephedrine and pseudoephedrine, will dilate swollen tissues allowing the sinuses to drain, points out Terry Willard, PhD, director of the Wild Rose College of Natural Healing in Calgary, Canada, and author of several books about herbs including *The Wild Rose Scientific Herbal* (Wild Rose College of Natural Healing). Ephedrine is classed as an adrenergic bronchodilator. It excites the sympathetic nervous system, depressing smooth muscle and cardiac muscle action, producing similar effects to those of epinephrine; however, it has a more prolonged effect than epinephrine, notes Willard.

Since *Ephedra* stimulates the nervous system, long-term use can cause adrenal exhaustion, according to Willard. Adding reishi mushroom and the herb licorice along with Vitamins B6 and C to your supplement regimen can help overcome this side effect, he notes.

It's important to remember that *Ephedra* is a strong central nervous system stimulant and shouldn't be used if you or your adult children have high blood pressure, diabetes or thyroid or heart disorders or pregnant, or if taking a monomine oxidase inhibitor (a type of antidepressant).

Eyebright *(Euphrasia officinale)*

Eyebright, or Euphrasia officinale, was used by ancient Greeks to treat eye infections. The name Euphrasia is derived from the Greek "euphrosyne" which means gladness, (the name of one of the three graces who was distinguished for her joy and mirth). It's believed the name was given to the plant because eyebright induced gladness by helping the patient to see. In the 14th century, eyebright was used to cure "all evils of the eye." In the eighteenth century, eyebright ale and tea were popular beverages.

Described by M. Grieve in *A Modern Herbal* as "an elegant little plant", eyebright grows two to eight inches tall and flowers from July to September with numerous small, white or purplish flowers variegated with yellow. Today, the United Plant Savers, an organization dedicated to protecting endangered medicinal plants, placed eyebright on their "to watch" list, meaning that it may soon be "at risk."

Eyebright contains tannins, quercitin, Vitamin C, rutin, essential fatty acids, the glycoside aucuboside, caffeic and ferulic acids, sterols, choline, some basic compounds and a volatile oil. There has been no significant scientific research into the merits of this "elegant little plant." None of the chemical components of eyebright have been associated with a significant therapeutic effect, and there are no controlled human studies to evaluate its effectiveness in the treatment of eye irritations. Yet it remains in high esteem among Western herbalists for its use as an eyewash to soothe burning or tired eyes. Eyebright has cooling and detoxifying properties that make it especially useful for inflammations, especially of the eyes and sinuses, notes Michael Tierra, CA, ND, author of *The Way of Herbs*:

"Compressions with a decoction of eyebright will give surprisingly rapid relief of redness, swelling and visual disturbances in eye inflammations."

Eyebright's astringent and antibiotic properties make it useful for cleansing the eyes and its function as an eyewash is due to its antimicrobial, volatile oil content and astringent tannins, according to Mark Pedersen in *Nutritional Herbology, A Reference Guide to Herbs*.

He goes on to say: "Eyebright's medicinal properties include antibacterial (due to the volatile oils) and astringent (due to the tannins) with a possible hypatonic (liver toning) action. It is a blood purifier that enhances liver function. "Chinese philosophy gives every part of the universe an opposite. The liver is the internal organ that matches the eye as an external organ of the body. Therefore, according to Chinese medicine, any herb that strengthens the liver must also strengthen the eye."

According to herbalist Ed Smith, medical herbalist and owner of HerbPharm in Williams, Oregon: "Use of eyebright does indeed benefit the eyes. The herb contains flavonoid pigments that specifically affect mucous membranes in the eyes and nasal passages. The flavonoids in eyebright are anti-inflammatory and stabilize mast cells, the lining in nasal passages. These cells make up the tissue that usually reacts to allergens."

"The use of eyebright can help break the allergy cycle, caused when you breathe in pollen and your body overreacts with burning eyes and runny nose. This inflammation increases your sensitivity to pollen, which then intensifies the inflammation. Use of eyebright can break this allergy cycle."

David Hoffmann author of *The Herbal Handbook*, calls

eyebright an excellent remedy for the problems of inflamed mucous membranes. The combination of anti-inflammatory and astringent properties makes it relevant in many conditions. Used internally, it is a powerful anticatarrhal (helps the body remove excess mucus), and may help relieve congestion. Best known for its use in eye irritations, it can relieve inflammations, stinging and weeping eyes, and is valuable in conjunctivitis.

While there are no known risks associated with eyebright, German studies suggest that 10 to 60 drops of eyebright tincture could cause side effects that include tearing, itching, redness and swelling of the eyelids. Varro Tyler, PhD, author of *The New Honest Herbal*, (Stickley), discourages topical eye applications of eyebright, especially of non-sterile homemade lotions, containing poorly known compounds.

You can purchase eyebright drops, combined with stinging nettle specifically created for children. However, check with your pediatrician or holistic practitioner to ensure it's the right solution for your child.

Stinging Nettles (Urtica dioica)

If you happen to brush up against an adult stinging nettle plant, it will probably make a lasting impression on you. The needle-like hairs of Urtica dioica will sting you like a swarm of fire ants, and you'll quickly develop a healthy respect for this potent plant.

Derived from the Anglo-Saxon word for "needle," the nettle has been regarded as a powerful medicinal herb for centuries. In 16th century England, nettle tea relieved many springtime maladies and was used as a tonic to purify blood, stimulate kidneys and stop internal bleeding. Around the third century BC, Hippocrates' Greek contemporaries prescribed nettle juice taken internally as an antidote to such plant poisons as hemlock and henbane. Roman soldiers flailed themselves with the stinging nettles in cold climates because the herb's sting warmed their freezing skin. Nettle sting is also a folk remedy for arthritis inflammation.

In the US, American Indian women believed drinking nettle tea during pregnancy strengthened the fetus, eased delivery and helped stop bleeding after childbirth. Nursing mothers used nettle tea to increase their milk production.

Today, nettles is recognized as high in Vitamin C and a rich source of chlorophyll. Constituents include histamine, formic acid, chlorophyll, glucoquinine, iron and Vitamin C. Nettles acts as an astringent, a diuretic and a tonic.

"Nettles are one of the most widely applicable plants we have." They strengthen and support the whole body", says David Hoffman.

In a 1990 randomized, double-blind clinical study reported in *Planta Medica: Journal of Medicinal Plant Research*, researchers noted that freeze-dried stinging nettles relieved allergy symptoms in over half of the participating patients. Indeed, 58percent of the participants taking two 300 mg capsules of freeze-dried Urtica dioica for one week experienced reduced symptoms of seasonal allergic rhinitis. (*Planta Medica* 1990 (56):44-47). James Duke, PhD and author of *The Green Pharmacy*, says: "We shouldn't be surprised that nettle does in fact help relieve allergy symptoms. For centuries, cultures around the world have used this herb to treat nasal and respiratory troubles including coughs, runny nose and chest congestion".

Stinging nettle's diuretic activity has been the subject of a number of German studies. One study in the early 80s found that nettle juice had a distinct diuretic effect on patients with heart problems. In 1989, German researchers Wagner et al, reported in *Planta Medica* that several fractions from nettles root showed anti-inflammatory effects in animal trials and stimulated human lymphocytes in vitro. In Germany, the herb is used in modern phyto-medicine for treatment of kidney infections, inflammation of the lower urinary tract and for treatment of renal gravel.

Toxic effects from drinking nettle tea have been recorded. These include: gastric irritation, burning sensation of the skin, edema and urine suppression. And according to Michael Castleman, author of *The Healing Herbs*, nettles stimulates uterine contractions in animal studies, and therefore, pregnant women should not use it internally.

Again, you can purchase stinging nettle, in combination with eyebright for your child. Please check with your pediatrician or holistic practitioner.

Elder (Sambucus nigra)

"The elder tree is a medicine chest by itself", notes herbalist David Hoffmann.

"There have been few scientific studies of elder's medicinal benefits, however elder leaves have been used traditionally for bruises, sprains and wounds, while elder flowers have been used to treat colds and flu", Hoffmann explains.

"They (elder flowers) may be used quite safely in any catarrhal (mucus) inflammation of the upper respiratory tract, such as hay fever and sinusitis," he notes.

A 1995 placebo-controlled clinical study reported in *The Journal of Alternative & Complementary Medicine* tested a standardized elderberry extract in 40 individuals suffering from flu symptoms. Researchers found a significant improvement in symptoms in 93 percent of cases within two days, versus six days for the control group. The researchers also documented anti-viral activity for the elderberry extract in vitro. They concluded that elderberry extract is active against influenza infections without adverse side effects.

"Inhibition of several strains of influenza virus in vitro and reduction of symptoms by an elderberry extract during an outbreak of influenza B in Panama". *Journal of Alternative & Complementary Medicine* (1995;1(4):361-369.)

The elder's constituents include flavonoids: rutin, isoquercitfrine and kampherol; tannins and essential oils, as well as Vitamins C and P found in the berries. Hoffmann lists the elder's actions as: diuretic, purgative, diaphoretic, anti-catarrhal and laxative.

An Echinacea and Goldenseal combination may also be effective in keeping the condition stable. Echinacea is anti-viral and Goldenseal is anti-bacterial, and soothes the mucous membranes of the throat and sinuses. Both herbs help to support immune response, which often becomes compromised due to prolonged allergic reaction. When used with other blood cleansers such as Red Clover, Sage, and Burdock, this combination cleanses the lymph and blood. It also clears toxic metabolites that result from the allergic response out of the system. An Echinacea and Goldenseal combination is also effective for treating, as well as preventing, sinusitis or actual sinus infection that often accompanies hay fever symptoms.

Licorice Root

Real licorice root, not the candy kind, is traditionally used to treat allergy and asthma. It also has a strengthening effect on the adrenal glands, which is weakened during the hay fever reaction. Licorice root extract may be taken during the hay fever season to treat, as well as lessen, the symptoms of allergy. In small doses, it is safe for children. Consult with your doctor on the amount to be given on a daily basis.

Astragalus

The last important herb is astragalus, the renowned Chinese botanical that strengthens the body's defensive or protective energy. It supports the body's ability to resist infections and other disease, and is used for its deep toning properties. Although astragalus does not directly treat hay fever and allergy symptoms, it may be taken one to two weeks per month during the hay fever and allergy seasons. Offer your child a cup of astrgalus tea made from the root. Have the root simmer in hot water for approximately 30 minutes then discard the root before drinking.

VITAMINS

Nutritionally, Pantothenic acid (Vitamin B-5) is often effective in the treatment of hay fever. Like Licorice, it helps to strengthen adrenal function, which is intimately involved with immune response. Dosages depend on the age of the child.

According to the US National Library of Medicine's dietary reference intake (DRI), dosages range from 1.7 milligrams per day to 5 mg per day.

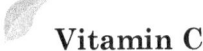

Vitamin C

Hay fever may also respond to Vitamin C. Preferably mineral ascorbate with bioflavonoids in a dose of 250 mg for a child four years old and up, two to four times daily between meals. For children under four, 100 mg should be enough. As always check with your pediatrician or holistic practitioner. The bioflavonoids are particularly effective, because they have an anti-inflammatory effect on the sinus cavity.

HOMEOPATHIC REMEDIES

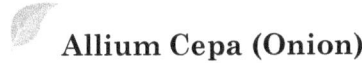

Allium Cepa (Onion)

This remedy is made from the red onion, so children who benefit from it will experience relief from symptoms, such as streaming nose with a burning discharge and watery, stinging eyes with bland secretion. They may also be relieved from violent sneezing and a tickling cough. This remedy usually comes in tablet or pellet form.

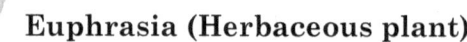

Euphrasia (Herbaceous plant)

A child who needs this remedy is suffering from eyes that are discharging, watery and stinging with bland secretions. They may also experience violent sneezing and a tickling cough.

Arsenicum (Arsenic)

Use arsenicum (in homeopathy, the arsenic is extremely diluted until there is little to no trace of it in the solution), when the mucus membranes of the child's eyes and nose are affected, and the secretions are extremely acrid. The nose produces a tin, watery discharge, but can also feel stuffed up, a similar feeling to the onset of a cold. He or she sneezes without relief.

Sabadilla (Plant)

This remedy will help ease continuous and violet sneezing and frustrating itching and tickling of the nose. One nostril may be blocked up while the other streams perhaps worsened by the smell of flowers. Your child's eyes burn and are watery.

ASTHMA: STATISTICS, CAUSES & NATURAL MANAGEMENT

Asthma is a commonly occurring condition, which can be serious and life threatening if not dealt with properly. According to the asthma society of Canada, it is a serious chronic lung disease affecting over 2.4 million people. Asthma affects all age groups and this includes approximately 15 percent of children. In Canada, asthma is one of the leading cause of admissions to hospitals and unfortunately, some 20 children and 500 adults will die from asthma. In fact, according to the lung association, 20 percent of Canadians, six million adults and children have a respiratory problem. The National Institutes of Health, WHO report, states that asthma is now a serious public health problem and affects over 100 million people worldwide.

In asthmatic conditions there is inflammation of the airways, or bronchi, which affects the way air enters and leaves the lungs, thereby disrupting breathing. When allergens or irritants come into contact with the inflamed airways, the already sensitive airways tighten and narrow, making it difficult for the person to breathe. As symptoms progress, it can lead to an asthma attack. Some of the changes in the bronchial tubes and airways that bring about these symptoms include: thick mucus production within the bronchial tubes, inflamed bronchial tubes becoming more swollen and/or broncho constriction, which is when the muscles around the bronchial tubes tighten, resulting in the airways narrowing. The symptoms associated with asthma differ from person to person. Most people experience severe coughing in the early morning hours or at night. The wheezing and tightening of the chest, plus other symptoms suffered by asthmatics, causes shortness of breath.

Over the past 20 years, there has been an increase in the prevalence of asthma in Canada. Clinical researchers are trying to ascertain why the increase. There is a correlation to urbanization with an increase in asthma. However, the risk is unclear since studies have not taken into account indoor allergens, although these have been identified as significant risk factors. The strongest risk factors are exposure, especially in infancy, to indoor allergens, i.e., mites, carpets, pets and a family history of asthma or allergies. Other important risk factors to consider include tobacco smoke, chemical irritants, perfumes, air spray products, mold, pollen, dust, drugs and respiratory infections. Even the weather, especially in colder months, stress and strenuous physical exercise can exacerbate asthma.

Currently, there is no cure, but there are medications and lifestyle changes that can help alleviate the symptoms so that one can lead a productive life. Many acute attacks among children can be prevented. Health Canada conducted a survey among school-aged children and found that 47 percent of children reported that household pets triggered or worsened their disease: 41 percent had a dog and 36 percent had a cat inside their home. Similarly, 54 percent of asthmatic children were exposed to second hand smoke, yet smoke was identified as worsening their asthma. Cigarette smoking is the single most prevalent cause of preventable illness and premature death in Canada. To educate the public on affects of cigarettes is crucial, and by reducing tobacco usage among the younger population, is the best hope for long-term reduction in lung cancer.

The best way to minimize the symptoms is to avoid the triggers. Changing bed and pillow coverings on a regular basis, avoiding mold, staying away from pets, and avoiding the outdoors during windy days are some of the lifestyle changes a person can make to eliminate the triggers.

To help manage asthma naturally, there are many vitamins, minerals, trace minerals and herbal supplements a child can use on a daily basis. Proper nutrition is important since asthma can be a symptom of food allergies. One must try to avoid fruit juices, nuts(peanuts) and milk, which are some of the most allergenic foods. Avoid monosodium glutamate(MSG), food additives(dyes, sulfites), shellfish, eggs and refined carbohydrates and chocolate since they provoke asthma in sensitive individuals.

- Vitamin C, an antioxidant, beneficial for the cells of the respiratory tract.
- Capsicum and Garlic capsules increase blood flow and immunity.
- Vitamin E, an anti-oxidant, inhibits formation of inflammatory compounds.
- Calcium/magnesium relaxes bronchial smooth muscle
- Chamomile is antispasmodic and a sedative, ideal for babies and children.
- Vitamin C and Zinc citrate lozenges strengthen immunity and soothes the throat.
- Ginkgo biloba improves circulation and helps increase blood flow to extremities.
- Bioflavonoids (quercetin, rutin) boost the immune system and is an antioxidant.
- Fish oils: Omega 3,6,9, Evening primose oil and essential fatty acids.
- B Vitamins are ideal for nervous system, stress.
- Multi-vitamins and minerals provide antioxidants, daily nutrients as supplements for overall energy and proper metabolism.

Remember asthma is a chronic condition and will require continuous medical attention and care. One must become proactive and follow these tips:

- Learn and educate yourself about asthma.
- Know what can trigger your child's asthma and avoid them.
- Learn how to use medications properly.
- Have a written asthma action plan.
- Work with a Certified Asthma Educator to learn about asthma control.
- Learn about natural approaches in early stages and build immunity naturally.
- Educate yourself on foods that causes allergies and eliminate.
- Introduce health choices, which includes fresh, organic fruits and vegetables.
- Implement stress-reduction techniques (Tai Chi, Yoga, Deep breathing exercises).
- Have a positive outlook in life.

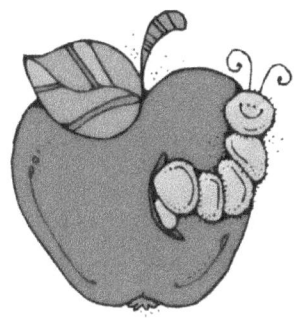

5 NUTRITIONAL TIPS

Excerpts from the book, *Children's Diet* were written in the early part of the century by Dr. Bircher Benner. The value of the following pages is for children ages two and up to 92. Some of the finest writings and nutritional counsels for children were written by him. He was the founder of a prestigious health spa in Switzerland.

Rather than attempting to duplicate the wisdom of the best authority in the field, Dr. Benner's thoughts are summarized in the following paragraphs.

Children require a natural, whole and non-artificial diet - a diet which God, nature and the forces of life have compounded and created..The wonderful, harmoniously attuned atomic and molecular structures, charged with light, the formations of air, water, life and spirit – these are designed as food.

The much extolled unnatural diet of the civilized nations is annoying like a worm at the very marrow of humanity. Without the careful example of adults and parents, the children's diet is not possible. Reverence for life, health and for the image of God created in all of us and in our infants, should prevent us from changing them arbitrarily and thoughtlessly before we incorporate them in our bodies? But we tear them to pieces and destroy them.

We have not considered that in doing so, we are also tearing to pieces and destroying the body, the bones, the teeth and the blood of our children, the future generation of mankind, and developing a barrier between the life that is within us and the Spirit.

The decline of the West begins in the degeneration of the diet of civilized nations. Social misery, spiritless politics are biological consequences of our physiological perversity. There is a relation between non-nutritious foods and health. Diet brings health only when all food factors are in the natural harmony with those who ingest them.

The harm done to our nutrients affects not only the constitution and the health of the individual, but also the basic cell nature, thereby its affect upon succeeding generations appear earlier and more seriously. Every population today, presents variations of individuals with varying basic cell natures. With similar manners of living, some remain apparently healthy, while others later fall victim to disease. Defective diet is to a large extent responsible for all this almost universal deterioration in health and of constitutional wellbeing.

The consumption of stimulants and intoxicants, lack of exposure to sunlight and ill-regulated living, add serious effects to deficiencies and their manifestations.

Inferiority of recent generations is often attributed to heredity – the immutable decree of destiny and a block to all attempts at curing. In reality, health regeneration is possible by removal of causes, and this to a great extent, especially in the early years of life, through corrections of errors in the composition, preparation and cooking of food.

Agriculture

The soil, upon which the food-giving light plants grow, becomes weakened through unsuitable soil treatment. This creates deficient foods. Animals, which provide our milk and meat, feeding on such soils, cannot create quality milk. The meat of such animals is remarkably less nutritious. Man, in turn, offers the effects of those deficiencies right through the chain of successive generations.

Artificial processing, manufacturing and preparing foods, disrupt the natural correlations of the food ingredients. For example, one simple food factor, separated from the whole and "refined" is, in that processed state, much less effective and very different from its natural association with the whole food.

The effects of violation of these laws, during the years of growth are more profound. The laws of diet hold good for children and adults alike.

Feeding Advice

Never force a child to drink milk, or to take any food, against his or her will. Force-feeding can associate eating in the child's mind with displeasure. To force solid foods too soon, is to ignore the baby's natural instinct.

Never take too lightly a baby's reactions to his or her foods. Learn to listen to your children. Babies and children have instincts with accurate guidelines to their needs. These instincts accurately tell them their body cannot use or tolerate certain foods. They resist or dislike those foods, or have digestive problems after eating or drinking them. They repulse or spit up unwanted solid foods from their mouth until the time when the body can handle them well.

Diet is health-creating in proportion to the degree of its content of all nutrients required by the body.

"Man thrives best on a moderate intake of foods, enough to cover his needs. This is possible only with a properly balanced diet and on the assumption that it is thoroughly masticated." - Russell H. Chittenden, American Physiologist

Vegetables

Well-chosen and prepared, alive vegetable foods are able to help heal many health disorders when other curative measures fail. Many animals build their bodies solely from vegetable proteins. Green leaves and plants contain valuable proteins. Greens provide a much better quality protein than milk, meat or many supplements. They add completeness to the imperfect proteins in seeds, grains, beans, lentils and peas.

Dried Fruits and Vegetables

Drying is a natural, acceptable form of food preserving. However, certain nutrients are lost by drying and storing. These foods are less complete and inferior to whole fresh foods. Dried foods should never exclude or take the place of fresh foods, if possible. Their role is to serve as seasonal stopgaps until fresh foods are available.

Vegetable powders and dried pulverized leaves are available at health food stores. These may contain parsley, radishes, tomatoes, spinach, beets, green beans, celery, carrots, leaks and herbs spices, etc. Mix them with other foods, soups, salads, etc.

Potatoes

The most nutritious portion of the potato is in the skin and in the flesh just under the skin. Its nutrients are lost mostly by over cooking. The skin protects and somewhat insulates the potato's flesh from the effects of excess heat. It prevents the leaching out of minerals in the starch.

Less food destruction or denaturing occurs by steaming in waterless cookers, or in a boiler in the bottom of which there is a small portion of water, than by boiling. Boiling in water to the point where the potato is soft enough to mash, destroys a lot of the potato food value. There is up to 50 percent more food value in a steamed potato than in a boiled potato. Potato seed sprouts contain a toxic substance.

Breads

The most nourishing breads are made from combinations of corn, rye, oats, millet or buckwheat. Canadian and American wheat is not as desirable a food as we have been conditioned to believe. What's marketed as "natural wheat" is man-made artificial strains of wheat. Their protein content is about one third the levels of natural wheat.

Their gluten content is five times greater than the original wheat. Just like mixing flower in water, this excess gluten leaves a glue in the intestines and thickens up the blood. It can seriously hamper blood circulation or make it sluggish.

Refined white flour is milled to death. A great number of essential ingredients are taken out. Minerals and vitamins are destroyed or extracted. Enriching flour puts back in a fraction of what has been taken out.

"An absence, a deficiency or a surplus of one or more of essential nutrient factors, causes injury to health. Of the many changes which occurred in the nature of food, none had such far-reaching and harmful influence on the health of people as those which affected the character of bread." - Dr. Drummond, Prof. of Biochemistry, London England

The word "enriched" flour or bread is grossly misleading. Natural, wholesome nutrients are extracted and replaced with chemical substitutes. Even if all the constituents of enriched bread correspond to government health laws, what is added is only a fraction of what has been extracted. The processed, refined vitamins and minerals additives that are replaced, are chemicals and unnatural. They are only fractions of the original vitamin/mineral complexes. They provide almost none of the body's health needs.

The more the bread is cooked, the harder the outer crust. The inner bread portion is more nourishing than the outer or crust layers. The greater the amount of crust the greater the need to chew. Dry bread crusts, or crisp foods, contribute little enamel hardness. Hardness depends on the nutrients and values of whole foods of the overall diet. However, chewing only soft bread can contribute to inferior tooth enamel. Crusts excite stomach glands to discharge unnecessary excesses of their digestive juices.

Cooking destroys bread nutrition wholeness. The common baking oven heats the inside of the bread up to temperatures of 350°F. This heat destroys food values and enzymes. It dextrinizes starches – turns starches into sugar-type substances. Dextrinized starches contain only a fragment of the food value of the original starch from which it is made.

White flour predisposes a child to allergies and to Vitamin B deficiency disease called 'Beriberi'. Storage of flours, even for short periods of time, diminishes their food value. Flours go rancid. Their oils are denatured by contact with air within two days. Grains ground into flour must be used for bread baking, as soon as possible after milling. Loaves, once cooked, can be safely stored in a freezer.

Food Mastication

Thorough mastication is important. All foods, but especially the starch foods, must be thoroughly masticated. If not properly chewed, foods will go down as chunks. These overload the stomach. It is much more difficult for the body to digest, utilize and be nourished by them.

Mastication increases the flow of saliva into the mouth and foods. Saliva is essential to thorough digestion, especially of starch and sugar foods. These, if not thoroughly mixed with saliva in the mouth, cannot digest further down in the digestive tract. They ferment. This causes harmful gas.

Cavities, pyorrhea and poor enamel hardness hamper the chewing capacity of many people. When chewing is poor, hard foods, such as carrots, cabbages, nuts, grains etc., need to be chopped finely or macerated through a blender.

Never dip breads or dough type foods in milk or coffee. The spreading of fat on breads interferes with the secretion of saliva essential to its good digestion. Buttering bread has some of this effect.

MOM & DAD...

- Develop good eating habits. Learn good nutrition. Select only the best, the freshest and most alive nutrients.
- Set the example in what you eat and how you live, feel and drink and think.
- Appreciate and try to never forget your children are special individuals. Try to treat them as such. For example, a father talking to his son: "Son, you are only a man, but son you are a man".
- In your own diets, include a variety of foods of high nutritional value as an example your children will follow.
- Do not compromise the quality of your foods by including convenient junk foods and foods lacking essential nutrients.
- Read labels carefully at the grocery and health stores.

To help you to better understand your child, and to provide you with the encouragement that comes through recognizing the signs of infant normality, I will include the following chart.

INFANT DEVELOPMENT

AGE	FEEDING SKILLS	REACTIONS
3-6 months	Tongue projects so that swallowing food is difficult Finger foods	
6-12 months	Uses hands Perceives size, shape, weight and texture. Eats by using tongue-lips. Chewing movements start. Reads facial expressions and gestures Takes juices and water from cup, but spills when cup is removed.	Very demanding of who feeds him/her
12-18 months	Grasps and releases, and fingers foods Grasps spoon; inserts it in dish; fills it poorly. Often turns spoons upside down Releasing of cup and spoon is poor.	Demands everything in sight at the table. Refuses milk from the bottle Loves an audience Frequently drops cup or spoon.
18-24 months	Decrease in appetite Feeds self	Becomes ritualistic Refusals –

	Drinks well from cup, but cup release is poor Turns spoon in mouth	preferences Easily distracted Tongue can lick chin
2-3 years	Drinks with small glass held with one hand Spoon is grasped between thumb and index finger and goes into mouth without turning Demands to eat – whole foods, between meal snacks; candy, when at home Considerable spilling Dislikes vegetables Food is most important part of his/her second birthday	Finicky and fussy eaters Spotless eaters, may demand to be fed Messy eater; refuses foods Goes on food jags Dawdles, ritualistic Dislikes food mixtures
3-4 years	Holds cup by handle Tilts head back to an empty cup Milk intake increases Pours from pitchers	Conforming, assertive Appetite becomes fair Asks for favorite foods

	Vegetables now accepted Uses a fork Now spills less/little Needs little assistance Chew foods more often	Is able to choose between alternatives A birthday cake is an important part of a 3rd birthday
4-5 years	Uses knife and fork with increasing ease Tilts cup to empty it	Assertive, lively mind Becomes more sociable Appetite – fair to good Food jags or strikes Reacts to incentives Eats to be like an adult Sets table Helps cooking

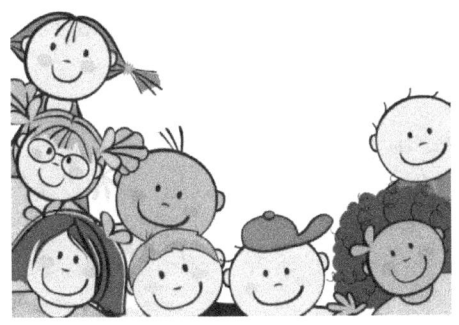

6 YOUR CHILD'S HAPPINESS

Everything in a child's life depends upon his or her health. Emotions, home, friends and happiness help create an environment conducive to optimal well-being and future happiness. Any considerable abnormality of body structure, becomes the source of feelings of inferiority.

A child's happiness depends greatly upon their nutritional and emotional contentment. If a food is satisfying, natural and well balanced, a child will be calm. It will sleep longer. It will be content – not nervous – not easily upset – not continually demanding attention. There will be less child tenseness and less upsetting the whole household.

Never forget to nourish a child with its most needed of all nutrients: tender, loving care. Apply tender, loving care through body touching, caressing words, smiles and songs in generous doses. Even use your tender loving care in the preparation and handling of foods.

States of Mind

The attitudes and mind conditioning impressed upon infants in the first three years of their lives remain with them and influence them physically, emotionally and mentally for their lifetime.

Minds and bodies are as strong, intelligent, vibrant, alive, capable and enthusiastic, as they are healthy, and these according to the amounts of quality nutrients they put into their bodies, minds and emotions. There is little difference in building human bodies than in building houses or motors. They all will be as excellent as the raw materials that go into building them.

Most babies, as they grow, who have been nourished and treated in ways indicated in these pages, almost inevitably succeed in being top "A" plus students, top athletes and eventually tops in the fields of work or the vocations they choose.

One wonders why parents will never tolerate inferior products or furniture in their homes or inferior products, or inferior gasoline in their automobiles, yet give not a moment's thought of filling their bodies, and the bodies of their children with useless, fast foods, junk foods and nonfoods and allow them to fill their minds with mindless and violent TV programs, and the art and music devoid of human emotions.

The above advice and cautions will be able to manage and control possibly up to 95 percent of all illnesses to which infants and young children are frequently prone.

`````
`````

A healthy child can mean a normal life for his or her parents.

- A life free of unusual worries and harassments.
- Free of being a slave to tyrannical whims and needs, every minute of the day.
- Normal, relatively undisturbed nights' sleep – at least after the first few months.
- Free of the worry that disease is always impending: tonsils will have to come out, periodic visits to the doctor are necessary, shots, antibiotics or drugs will be needed.

PARENTS, YOU ARE ALL YOUR CHILDREN HAVE!

LOOK AFTER *YOU* WELL

KEEP JOY IN YOUR LIFE

REFERENCES

1. Earache MedlinePlus. Internet (Cited on Nov 22th, 2013): http://www.nlm.nih.gov/medlineplus/ency/article/003046.htm

2. Ely JW, Hansen MR, Clark EC. Diagnosis of ear pain. *Am Fam Physician*. 2008;77(5):621-628.

3. Natural Health Products Directorate Monograph: Garlic. Internet (Cited Nov. 24th, 2013):http://www.hc-sc.gc.ca/dhp-mps/prodnatur/applications/licenprod/monograph/mono_echinacea_purpurea_e.html

4. Natural Health Products Directorate Monograph: Vitamin C. (Internet) (Cited Nov. 24th, 2013):http://www.hc-sc.gc.ca/dhpmps/prodnatur/applications/licenprod/monograph/mono_vitamin_c_e.html

5. Natural Health Products Directorate Monograph: Echinacea purpurea. (Internet) (Cited Nov. 24th, 2013): http://www.hcsc.gc.ca/dhpmps/prodnatur/applications/licenprod/monograph/mono_echinacea_purpurea_e.html

6. *Everybody's Guide to Homeopathic Medicine.* (Internet): (Cited on Nov. 23, 2013) http://www.homeopathic.com/Articles/Using_homeopathy_for_ailments/Homeopathic_Medicines_for_Earaches.html

7. Live Science (Internet): Cited August 2016) http://www.livescience.com/51640-b5-pantothenic-acid.html

8. The Clark's and Young's Rule: (Internet) (Cited: August 10, 2016) http://www.pharmacytechstudy.com/dosecalculation.html#clark

Thank you, Pixel Worlds, krwz of Vector clipart and Olga Matushkina for the use of your images.

ABOUT THE AUTHOR

Dr. Elvis Ali is highly respected for his work in Naturopathic Medicine. Dr. Elvis, as he is affectionately known, has been in private practice for over 30 years, specializing in Chinese and sports medicine and nutrition. With impressive credentials - Bachelor of Science, majoring in Biology, Licensed Acupuncturist, Doctorate in Naturopathic Medicine; Mind/Body Medicine at Harvard Medical School, Diploma in Homeopathic Medicine - he lectures internationally, written several books and appeared on radio and television shows. His passion lies in empowering people by educating them on complementary health and wellness, and non-intrusive options.